ON DOCTORAL EDUCATION IN NURSING:

The Voice of the Student

ON DOCTORAL EDUCATION IN NURSING:
The Voice of the Student

Dona Rinaldi Carpenter, EdD, RN, CS
Sharon Hudacek, EdD, RN, CS

NLN Press • New York
Pub. No. 14-6703

Copyright © 1996
National League for Nursing Press
350 Hudson Street, New York, NY 10014

ISBN 0-88737-670-3

Library of Congress Cataloging-in-Publication Data

Carpenter, Dona Rinaldi.
    On doctoral education in nursing : the voice of the student / Dona
Rinaldi Carpenter, Sharon Hudacek.
        p.   cm.
    Includes bibliographical references.
    ISBN 0-88737-670-3
    1. Nursing—Study and teaching (Graduate)—United States.
    2. Doctor of philosophy degree—United States.   I. Hudacek, Sharon.
    II. Title.
    RT75.C37   1996
    610.73'071'173—dc20   95-46194
                                                                    CIP

This book was set in Bembo by Eastern Composition, Inc., Binghamton, New York.
Northeastern Press, in Waymart, Pennsylvania was the printer and binder. Nancy Jeffries
was the editor and designer. Cover design by Lauren Stevens.

Printed in the United States of America

Contents

Foreword

THIS BOOK REPRESENTS our work related to issues in doctoral education in nursing that began in 1989 when, in a qualitative research course, Dr. Patricia Munhall asked us to explore the meaning of doctoral education in nursing using different qualitative methods. The small scale phenomenological investigation we conducted led to the expansion of the study after the course, development of a quantitative tool based on the qualitative data, and a national study that resulted in more than 400 narrative responses from doctoral students throughout the country. These responses were reviewed, topically organized and are presented in this book along with pertinent literature related to some of the most significant issues in doctoral education in nursing. Additionally, quantitative data from the accompanying questionnaire is also included in relevant categories.

ABOUT THE STUDY

The study results included in this book were sparked by the realization that students in DNS, EdD, and PhD doctoral nursing programs had not been collectively surveyed about their beliefs and views on doctoral education. The study explored, from a student perspective, views on such areas as research preparation, curriculum content, critical thinking, mentorship, and collegiality within DNS, EdD, and PhD programs in nursing.

Doctoral programs listed in the Sigma Theta Tau International listing from 1991 were included in the study. Twenty students in each of the 54 programs nationwide were asked to complete a questionnaire that included three parts. *Part I* was a 117-millimeter continuum with ends defined as "agree" and "disagree." Students were asked to respond in this section by marking a line across the continuum that intersected the matched belief. Data collected requested information about the influence of doctoral education on personal and professional growth; excellence as a practitioner, researcher, educator, and/or administrator; and decision making, critical thinking and problem solving abilities. Other questions requested the student to differentiate between degree types in terms of research preparation, rigor, mentorship, peer support, and experiences with doctorally prepared faculty.

Part II of the questionnaire elicited narrative comments and qualitative data about doctoral education in nursing. The responses of the participants in the section of the study have been integrated throughout the book with selected narrative comments included verbatim. Finally, *Part III* of the questionnaire included demographic data about the participants in the study.

Content validity for the tool was established by requesting doctorally prepared nurses to review and critique the tool. Twelve individuals voluntarily agreed to review and critique the survey. Five faculty held EdDs as their highest degree, five were PhD prepared and two were graduates of DNS programs (all nursing doctorates). The final draft included revisions and suggestions from the expert panel.

HIGHLIGHTS OF KEY FINDINGS ADDRESSED IN THE BOOK

The study results revealed a great deal about students' beliefs and experiences in doctoral education. The details of the study have been integrated through the various chapters in the book. The highlights of the study are as follows:

1. Participants believe that doctoral education prepares one to be an excellent researcher and that research is the primary focus of any program—PhD, EdD, DNS.

2. The ability to write in a scholarly manner and publish is clearly enhanced for all students in doctoral education.
3. Research background in quantitative analysis is emphasized over qualitative analysis.
4. The role preparation students are focused on is research, with a second component that is either (in order of preference) educator, practitioner, or administrator.
5. Mentorship by faculty and networking with other students are viewed as essential components to doctoral education.
6. The majority of students believe that dissertation courses prepare them for their own individual research.
7. Students were more accepting of diversity in doctoral degree programs rather than favoring one degree.

Nurse educators are frequently asked by potential doctoral students to describe the educational process for nurse doctorates and to cite similarities and differences among the three degree types in nursing. Doctoral students should be advised about programmatic choices in order to attain the best "fit" between program type and their own educational and career goals. The data from this study provides information for doctoral students about the experiences and views of students already engaged in the doctoral education process and relates these narrative experiences to relevant literature.

CHAPTER HIGHLIGHTS

Chapter 1 provides the reader with an overview of the history of doctoral education in the United States and leads into a discussion of the historical evolution of the doctorate in nursing. The reader is also provided with a summary of the annual forums on doctoral education which are very helpful in providing a context within which to view the current status of doctoral education in nursing. Included as well are anecdotes from early nursing leaders regarding doctoral preparation.

Chapter 2 addresses program choices available to doctoral students. An overview of the degrees available, specifically in nursing, is initially provided along with the option of earning a doctorate in another field and the implications for professional nursing. This chapter is organized around a comprehensive review of available literature, and the quantitative as well as qualitative data obtained in the study reported and integrated throughout the book.

Chapter 3 lends focus to curricular issues in doctoral education as they currently exist and are addressed in the literature as well as the narrative comments of students participating in the study. This chapter is particularly helpful in sorting out differences, which are minimal, and similarities among doctoral curriculums.

Chapter 4 addresses the concept of mentoring and the central role that this experience plays in the doctoral education process. Key narrative comments related to students' experiences with the mentoring process are integrated throughout the chapter and related to literature addressing the importance of the mentoring experience across interdisciplinary lines.

Chapter 5 discusses the important concept of networking and the benefits experienced by students as they set up their support system and resources at this highest level of academic preparation. The networking that occurs in doctoral education leads to life-long relationships that may be both personal and professional.

Chapter 6 provides insightful information about the research expected at the doctoral level and the trends that have been established in the topics and methods used by doctoral students in selected dissertations. *Appendix A* complements this chapter with a listing of selected doctoral dissertations completed over the past four years.

Commitment to the doctoral education process requires much personal investment on the part of the student. *Chapter 7* reviews pertinent literature related to commitment and incorporates student concerns regarding commitment to doctoral education as well as family and work responsibility.

Chapter 8 is in some ways an extension of the topics addressed throughout the book. Obstacles that impact students throughout the doctoral education process are presented through frank comments of study participants.

The concluding *Chapter 9* addresses perhaps the most significant experience of the doctoral education process: that of personal and professional growth. This chapter ties together the central components of doctoral education—curriculum, role preparation, research, networking, and mentoring—as they impact on the individual's growth at work and in their everyday lives.

The book shares with the public the important aspects of doctoral education as voiced by over 400 doctoral students across the nation. Their voices have echoed much about what we hope for the future of nursing and for doctoral education. The incorporation of verbatim narrative comments throughout this book was done with the sole purpose of allowing others to hear about doctoral education through the voices of those actually engaged in the process. This book culminates our own need to know more about what other students are experiencing in doctoral education and ends a long search to find meaning in and validate our own experiences as doctoral students.

This book could not have been prepared without the help of our research assistants at the University of Scranton: Dawn Cramer, Jeanine Gannon, Susan Heim and Kerry Grundy. They spent their time helping us search the literature and compile references that both support and call into question many of the issues facing doctoral education in nursing today. Thanks are also extended to all the study participants who gave their valuable time to write reams of notes about their doctoral education experiences. We know that their efforts took commitment, and their dedication will help to advance professional nursing. Finally, we owe many thanks to our families and friends who have supported us throughout this endeavor and have once again accepted the fact that we are working full time during our vacations and have helped us throughout the six years we have been working on this project. To Vito, Elaine, Kay, Deb, Lisa, Loraine, Lynn, and Diane we say thank you for your help, support, and friendship. To Stephen and Brian, we promise that one morning we will sleep in, have a leisurely cup of coffee, and you won't find us at the computer at 6 A.M. To Stephen Jr., Chas, Emily, and Brian Jr., we love you!

CHAPTER ONE

The History of Doctoral Education in Nursing

INTRODUCTION

IN THIS CHAPTER we briefly review historical antecedents of doctoral education in America as well as discuss the historical development of doctoral education in nursing. Having a sense of how doctoral education came to be in America, and then, how doctoral education developed specifically in nursing, is important to all the discussions that follow. Issues that surround doctoral education in nursing today, and student experiences with doctoral education, are connected to our past and will influence the direction of doctoral education in the future.

Doctoral education in nursing is a timely as well as important topic for the profession. Discussions regarding the type of degree program most appropriate for the nursing profession continue, and the valuing of the Doctor of Philosophy (PhD) in nursing is evident throughout the literature. The fact remains, however, that nursing continues to prepare individuals at the doctoral level with varying degrees: the Doctor of Education (EdD), Doctor of Nursing Science (DNS), and the Doctor of Philosophy. The Doctor of Philosophy degree remains the most popular. The reason for this is probably related to historical antecedents of the evolution of this degree rather than actual differences in course requirements and preparation.

THE EARLY BEGINNING OF
DOCTORAL EDUCATION

The doctorate as an earned degree originated in Europe during the Middle Ages. Yale University had the distinction, in 1861, of being the first American institution to award the Doctor of Philosophy degree (Matarazzo & Abdellah, 1971). Approximately 60 years later, the first doctorate in nursing was available.

The earliest universities to develop doctoral education emerged during the Middle Ages in Paris and Bologna. During that time, doctoral preparation indicated that individuals in possession of a doctoral certificate were granted membership in the professors' guild. As doctoral education developed, teaching became a focus and the title of doctor conveyed full right to teach at any university without further examination (Malden, 1835). Licensing to teach later became the responsibility of clergy as well as professors. The approval of the Catholic Church was also at one time required for authorization to grant degrees (Marriner-Tomey, 1990).

Early American higher education limited itself to baccalaureate-level study. Graduate-level study developed in response to the influence of the German university. The German university system trained teachers, scholars, and civil servants. University professors were researchers who taught all their students with the same goal in mind; students were expected to be candidates for the doctorate. University professors and teachers in secondary schools were to earn PhDs (Nichols, 1967). Although Americans were returning from Germany with the doctorate in the 1820s, the first American PhD, awarded by Yale University, was introduced almost 40 years later. Johns Hopkins University was the first American university to develop based on the German model and began awarding the doctorate in 1876 (Spurr, 1970).

Adoption of the German university model in America was difficult for a number of reasons. Graduate faculty were not recruited. As a result, faculty who were not academically prepared assumed extra work for a higher level of education for which they were not ready. Furthermore, the organizational structure of American higher education which used credit hours as the measure of degree requirements presented a major obstacle. In contrast, German universities used major examinations to determine the awarding of degrees and were less formal about lecture periods than American universities (Veysey, 1973).

The German idea of a doctoral dissertation was a published, publicly defended contribution to knowledge and soon became the hallmark of the American PhD. In 1896, the Federation of Graduate Clubs recommended minimum requirements for the PhD which included: attainment of a baccalaureate degree; at least two years of graduate study with one year on the campus of the institution conferring the degree; adequate examination; and acceptable theses of original research (Spurr, 1970). The Association of American Universities was founded in 1900 to set uniform standards for the PhD which included such issues as residency and language requirements.

After World War I, the number of doctorates awarded increased significantly, and American higher education saw the extension of the PhD to professional fields. By 1940, the PhD was being awarded in agriculture, business, education, engineering, home economics, journalism, library science, nursing and social work (Berelson, 1960). This extension of the PhD into professional fields caused additional controversy in American higher education and the debate over whether the PhD should be awarded for professional study began. In 1920, Harvard awarded the doctorate in education, but it was the EdD rather than the PhD. Harvard now awards both the EdD and PhD in education but many universities continue to award only the EdD as the highest degree in education. And so the controversy over degree type began. Berelson (1960) noted "The exceptional regard that exists for the PhD in academic circles, where presumably most persons know better, has never been fully explained" (p. 39).

From 1900 to World War I, universities in the United States began looking at setting standards for the PhD. The National Association of State Universities recommended that a minimum of three years of post-graduate study be required for the PhD in 1908 and

standards were also set during this time for residency, language requirements, and dissertation requirements (Marriner-Tomey, 1990).

After World War I, the PhD was being awarded more frequently
and controversy developed over whether or not the PhD should be
awarded for professional study. According to Marriner-Tomey
(1990):

> Harvard awarded the EdD in 1920 but later awarded only the EdD
> as the highest degree in education. Several universities award only
> the EdD as the highest degree in education, while others award only
> the PhD in education. Still others grant both degrees. This pattern
> exists in other professional fields. In general, professions have sought
> the PhD as their highest degree (p. 134).

The fact that the PhD has been sought as the highest degree may be
related to historical antecedents. As other professions emerged—for
example, law, philosophy, medicine, and theology—emphasis was
placed on maintaining their professional significance. In these disciplines the professional doctorate is considered to have equal or
higher status than a research degree (Marriner-Tomey, 1990). Because other professionals have modeled their doctorates after the arts
and science PhD, providing a mixture of theory and technique, professional doctorates do tend to be indistinguishable from the PhD
(Marriner-Tomey, 1990).

THE BEGINNING OF DOCTORAL PREPARATION
FOR NURSES

Since the early part of the century nurses have been planning for
and developing doctoral education in nursing. It is only during the
last ten to fifteen years, however, that the most significant increase
in the number of programs has occurred. Among the most significant factors responsible for the development of doctoral education
for nurses were national industrialization, the pressures of war, demand by the public for higher education, and the feminist movement. Then as now, doctoral education was viewed as critical to the

preparation of future educators, researchers, and administrators (Pa-rietti, 1979).

In 1960, only four doctoral programs in nursing existed; by 1980, the number had grown to 21. In 1995, there are 59 doctoral programs in nursing. The majority of the programs are for the PhD, followed by the DNS degree. Teachers College continues to offer the only EdD in nursing. Edith S. Bryan was the first American nurse to earn a PhD in psychology and counseling from Johns Hopkins University in 1927 (American Nurses' Foundation, 1969).

Prior to the 1960s, doctoral education in nursing occurred in settings with the specific goals of preparing educators (EdD). In the early sixties, professional nurse doctoral programs developed (DNS). Bridging the generation and transmission of knowledge with the practice domain has always been a central issue for doctoral education, and thus the evolution of different degrees.

The first program to offer a doctoral degree in nursing was established at Teachers College, Columbia University in 1924. The *EdD (Doctor of Education)* was granted to nurses preparing to teach at the college level. Teachers College was at the forefront of nursing education and designed a program that focused on both the educational and nursing needs of leaders in the profession. "Teachers College is the only American institution to combine a nursing and education degree, in the form of two programs: in curriculum and nursing instruction, and in administration of education" (Gorney-Fadiman, 1981, p. 662).

The first *PhD (Doctor of Philosophy)* program in nursing was established in 1934 at New York University. The University of Pittsburgh followed in the 1950s with its PhD program in Maternal and Child Nursing. The University of Pittsburgh program was the first to emphasize the importance of clinical research for the advancement of nursing knowledge. PhD programs are considered to be primarily research-oriented in their focus, ultimately preparing nurses for intellectual inquiry that will develop the science of nursing practice (Werley & Leske, 1988).

A third program model, the *DNSc (Doctor of Nursing Science)*, was developed at Boston University and was based on the generation of nursing theory as the focal point of a practice discipline. This professional practice doctorate was promoted as the terminal degree for nursing because many nursing leaders believed that the four-year baccalaureate degree was not sufficient to prepare a nurse for the kind of independent practice needed by health care consumers. With a focus on the concepts of autonomy and independent practice, promoting the professional doctorate or the doctorate of nursing science was viewed as the means to an advanced educational base and improved professional status for nursing.

While all three program models originally were different, distinguishing program types has become muted. As doctoral education in nursing has developed, differences of opinion have arisen regarding how to proceed with the development of these programs. These differences of opinion regarding program type and curricular emphasis have been addressed at the annual doctoral forums discussed later in this chapter. In an effort to ensure quality education at the doctoral level, the implementation of new programs has proceeded with caution and precision. The 1950s also saw a dramatic upgrading of educational preparation for nurses with the federal government providing fiscal support for higher education here (Marriner-Tomey, 1990).

By the early 1960s, the goals and objectives of the nursing doctorate still had not been clearly delineated. With little agreement among nursing leaders on the topic, some argued that more deliberation and critical consideration of all aspects of program development were required (Elkins, 1960). At the same time, other nursing leaders believed that nursing was obligated to develop programs in doctoral education to create new knowledge through basic research on the doctoral level. Others suggested that nurses enroll in established programs in the natural and social sciences until a theoretical framework for nursing science based on substantive content in nursing was more effectively defined (Hassenplug, 1966).

In the early 1960s, there were at least four options for nurses seeking a doctorate: (1) the EdD, the professional degree in education and most commonly held by the few nurses with doctorates at that time; (2) the PhD in a cognate discipline which was encouraged by the Nurse-Scientist Graduate Training Program; (3) a professional degree exclusively for nursing (DNS); and (4) a PhD in nursing. Nurses prepared with doctorates in education or PhDs in other disciplines brought the nursing profession to a point where doctoral programs in nursing were possible (Matarazzo & Abdellah, 1971).

In an analysis of doctoral education in nursing, Grace (1978) identified three stages of development for nursing. Initially, there were *functional specialists*. During this period (1924–1959), doctoral degrees were earned primarily in the field of education. Nurses were prepared as teachers or administrators with a focus on role preparation—a trend consistent with how doctoral education had been developing in other professional disciplines. This phase reflected nursing's first efforts at doctoral education for the profession.

Schools of education provided an environment receptive to a practice discipline and focused on methods of teaching. However, primary focus was not granted to the substantive content of nursing per se, an issue which would later become central to doctoral preparation in nursing. Nurses studied teaching/learning theories, curriculum development, and teaching/evaluation methodologies. Research was directed toward education issues and not on building a knowledge base for nursing (Grace, 1989).

During the second developmental stage (1960–1969), a majority of nurses earned doctorates in scientific disciplines related to nursing. Nurses teaching at the college level now gained their doctorates in related disciplines such as anthropology, psychology, or sociology thus increasing the options available for nurses seeking doctoral education. According to Grace (1978), factors contributing to the increase in the number of doctorally prepared nurses at this time included: (1) development of doctoral programs in nursing; (2) support by special pre-doctoral research fellowships through the division of nursing; and (3) availability of faculty adequately prepared to implement doctoral programs in nursing. Issues that emerged here continue to impact on the evolution of doctoral education in nursing, and included: What is the essential nature of professional nursing? What is the substantive knowledge base of professional nursing? What kind of research is important for nursing as a knowledge discipline and as a practice discipline? How can the scientific base of nursing knowledge be identified and expanded? (Murphy, 1981). These questions were directly related to nursing's efforts to be recognized as a profession and continue to be debated even today.

One very important issue that was and is central to the ongoing discussion on doctoral education programs in nursing relates to reaching some agreement on its substantive content. Many nursing leaders had been doctorally prepared in the field of education and others in a variety of scientific disciplines. Each program type had instilled in the student traditions specific to the profession. Nursing leaders were bringing what they had learned in their doctoral programs to discussions about what type of doctorate would be appropriate for nursing. According to Grace (1989):

> Those coming from the natural sciences had been trained in a research-mentorship process in which research is learned through doing. Those trained in behavioral science fields were familiar with mastering a body of theoretical knowledge, learning independent research under the guidance of faculty researchers (Grace, 1989, p. 266).

The third and current stage of development was described by Grace (1978) as *doctorates in and of nursing*. During the 1970s, the educational preparation of nurses at the doctoral level was more specifically related to the discipline of nursing and was the result of an integration of related scientific fields into that of nursing. Newly established doctoral programs then offered the PhD and DNS degrees. Clearly the profession was struggling with the question of whether doctoral preparation should be clinically or research oriented.

Grace (1989) noted that "instead of increased differentiation as doctoral programs proliferated in the 1970s and early 1980s, the trend was for structure and content to become remarkably similar" (p. 267). Doctoral programs in nursing also were cast in the mold of the "research doctorate." These trends have significantly influenced the development of doctoral education in nursing. The results of the research study on doctoral education reported in this book concur with the trends Grace noted. According to Grace (1989):

> Many of these newly graduated doctorally prepared nurses, knowledgeable of the requirements for promotion and tenure and critical of their mentors, are setting their own research as a top priority, with clinical teaching, administration, and public service as much lower priorities (p. 267).

These patterns continue today making it ever more crucial to continue to evaluate and refine the direction of doctoral education in nursing.

CURRENT STATUS OF DOCTORAL EDUCATION IN NURSING

The nursing profession must clarify its need for doctorally prepared leaders. The fact remains that nursing is a practice discipline comprised of much diversity. Other practice disciplines such as psychology and education look at students in terms of those who possess the personality characteristics to be expert practitioners and those who would do better in a research track. Grace (1989) emphasized:

> Clinicians demonstrate integrative and holistic thinking patterns while researchers tend to be reductionist in their thought processes. Although both patterns of thinking are highly valued in the field, it is accepted that different individuals are more appropriately placed in one track over another. Rarely is the attempt made for an individual to be a master of both basic research and practice. It is acknowledged that the field of psychology needs both experimental and clinical psychologists and that the experimental psychologist needs a beginning understanding of principles of treatment and vice versa. However, in nursing we tend to adopt the position that one person

should be able to be all things and that the doctorally prepared nurse should be both a skilled basic researcher and an able practitioner (p. 268).

If you have been in the profession for any length of time, you become familiar with who is "good" at what. For example, while some faculty are excellent in research, other faculty are excellent in practice. In this light, very intelligent nurses who should be doing research are at the bedside trying to practice, an area that may not be a strength. Can you have both an expert researcher and practitioner?—perhaps. However, it is time for nursing to understand individual strengths—research, practice, or education—and to capitalize upon them. Specifically, we need different preparation for different leadership roles in nursing. We should enable individuals to make the most important contributions to the profession they are capable of, and reward them accordingly.

In 1971, a conference was held with nursing leaders to address future directions of doctoral education for nursing. This initial conference was important to the development of doctoral education in nursing and resulted in conferences that continue to this day. At this first conference, the central question asked was: what type of doctoral preparation for nurses should we have for the next decade and for the future (Murphy, 1981)?

Three doctoral degree types in nursing continue to exist and the debate over whether there should be one degree, the PhD, or a mix continues. Although a clear trend toward the PhD has been established, nursing must, as suggested, continue to examine the practice of attempting to prepare all leaders for all things. As criteria for evaluating doctoral programs also are established and upgraded, diversity in preparation comes to the fore. The goals of doctoral preparation must be clear, looking toward the establishment of a community of scholars who are capable of advancing nursing's research agenda and practice issues. As Leininger (1974) noted, doctoral education should produce scholars who are open minded, seek the ideas of others, and draw upon them to refine their own knowledge. The enthusiasm of doctorally prepared nurses for their own special knowledge should excite and stimulate those individuals whose careers and lives they influence.

A CHRONOLOGICAL LOOK AT THE ANNUAL FORUMS ON DOCTORAL EDUCATION IN NURSING

Since 1977, national conferences on doctoral education in nursing have monitored programmatic changes, planned for, implemented, and evaluated doctoral curricula. Initiated in 1977, the annual Forums on Doctoral Education in Nursing encouraged faculty members in established doctoral programs to exchange ideas. Debate has centered on issues in doctoral education, including projected needs in the curricula, with assessments on what has been achieved in doctoral education. In 1977, thirteen (13) doctoral programs were in existence, now there are 59. To date eighteen "national conferences" also called "forums" have been held throughout the country to discuss future tasks for educators, administrators, practitioners, and all those involved in the education of nurse doctorates.

In 1977, there were three broad conference goals: (1) feasibility, (2) purpose, and (3) implementation. The *feasibility* and need for nurses to attain doctoral education was rather moot at the time, considering that only 60 nurses per year were graduating with doctoral degrees. There was another concern, however, and a bit more practical: if nursing academics did not respond and provide adequate programs on the doctoral level, nurses would largely seek other fields and degrees outside nursing. The *purpose* for program development also offered interesting dialogue: "What labels do we affix to that program? What credential is to be borne by the graduate?" Two degree tracks were discussed: the professional doctorate for scholarly nursing practice and the PhD for research and theory development. An analogy was then made to the entry level debate and titling issues on the doctoral level. Nurse leaders were cautioned about the implementation of new programs while sharing concerns about the intensity of programs, structure, and the qualifications of students admitted. Also reviewed was the issue of accreditation.

Should the National League for Nursing (NLN), or The American Association of Colleges of Nursing (AACN), undertake this matter or leave doctoral education out of the context of accreditation altogether? Such questions provoked much important thought on doctoral education with forums continuing today.

In the remainder of this chapter, we will thus provide an overview of each forum held to date to more clearly understand our past as well as our present and future development in doctoral education. A topical overview of theoretical, curricular, support, resource and other pragmatic issues specifically addressed at each forum follows.

CONFERENCE HIGHLIGHTS

The first national conference in doctoral education prompted educators throughout the world to examine the *goals and issues confronting doctoral programs and the future of such programs*. Styles (1977) addressed three specific areas that educators must consider: "issues, questions, and tasks." Many other aspects of doctoral education were detailed: resources, faculty, dissertation requirements, and the nature of the content being delivered in these curricula (Proceedings of the 1977 Forum on Doctoral Education in Nursing).

Place: University of Pennsylvania School of Nursing
Date: June 23–24, 1977
Topics:
  1. Doctoral Education in Nursing: The Current Situation in Historical Perspective.
  2. Theoretical and Pragmatic Issues Related to the Goals of Doctoral Education in Nursing.
  3. Faculty Resources.
  4. Qualifications for Student Admission and Retention.
  5. Program Design.
  6. Nursing Course Content.

(*continued*)
  7. Financial Resources.
  8. Doctoral Education in Nursing: Future Directions from
     Current Experiences.

In 1978, discussion in the doctoral education arena focused on *program type*. The professional doctorate nurse preparation at Case-Western Reserve University and related admission requirements, learning opportunities, and characteristics of the Nurse Doctorate graduate were detailed. Three programs of study were reviewed: the Doctor of Nursing, which focused on Inquiry Care/Generalists Practice; the Master of Science in Nursing, with a focus on Care/Advanced Practice Inquiry; and the Doctor of Philosophy, focusing on Inquiry and preparing a nurse researcher. The practice-oriented doctorate or Nursing Science degree (DNS) was defined. The DNS at the University of Alabama was detailed in terms of philosophy, purpose, and objectives. The research doctorate or PhD was also defined by several nurse leaders as allowing for the development of new bodies of knowledge specific to the study of nursing. The NYU Rogerian model was detailed as an example. Future developments in nursing were forecasted, some of which included the expansion to home health, health teaching, and HMOs as the major forces influencing the hospital industry (Proceedings of the 1978 Forum on Doctoral Education in Nursing). A list of papers presented at the 1978 forum and a summary of group discussions follows.

Place: Rush University College of Nursing
Date: June 29 and 30, 1978
Topics:
  1. Doctor of Nursing Program: The Professional Doctorate
     in Nursing.
  2. The Professional Doctorate in Nursing from the
     Viewpoint of Nursing Science.

(*continued*)
   3. The Research Doctorate in Nursing.
   4. Future Developments in Nursing.
   5. Towards a Cooperative Venture in Program Evaluation
      of Doctoral Programs in Nursing.

In 1979, discussion involved *identifying the clinical content of nursing, quality in doctoral dissertations,* and *discussions on the doctorally prepared nurse in the scientific community.* The clinical component was viewed as just emerging. Attributes of high quality dissertations were elaborated upon, including the psychological, social and structural processes involved in completing such a dissertation. Conditions conducive to quality and dissertation dilemmas were described. Characteristics of the researcher and personal "scholarliness" were detailed, such as willingness to support one's conviction, accuracy, and integrity (p. 42). At the time, 22 doctoral programs were in existence and 18 consented to participate in a study on assessing the status of each program. Finally, a discussion on nursing and the behaviors that restrict nurses in the scientific community were offered. Suggestions were then given on how to strengthen the role of science in nursing and ultimately socialize nurses in this endeavor (Proceedings of the 1979 Forum on Doctoral Education in Nursing).

Place: Jack Tar Hotel, San Francisco, California
Date: June 28–29, 1979
Topics:
   1. Defining the Clinical Content of Nursing.
   2. An Analytical Model of Quality in Nursing Doctoral
      Dissertations.
   3. Cooperative Program Evaluation Project in Doctoral
      Education in Nursing.
   4. Preparing Doctorates in Nursing to Participate in the
      Scientific Community.

Three domains of nursing science set the stage for the 1980 conference: principles that govern life processes, well-being, and optimum functions of human beings; patterning of human behavior and interaction with the environment in critical life situations; and concern with processes by which positive changes in health status are affected. "Wholeness" and manifestations of wholeness were considered along with sub-concepts, such as energy fields and rhythmic phenomena. The principle of "complementarity" was described within the construct of patterns and health. Clinical studies on patterning (e.g., "Patterning of Sleep and Respiration During Sleep") were presented along with Leininger's "Caring and Caring Lifestyles" model. According to Leininger, caring was the central focus for nursing and doctoral research. World forces influencing the need for caring in nursing and a transcultural report of an ethnoscience investigation were offered. Finally, a report of the cooperative program evaluation project focusing on doctoral education in nursing was offered (Proceedings of the 1980 Forum on Doctoral Education in Nursing).

Place: Wayne State University College of Nursing
Date: June 26–27, 1980
Topics:
1. Principles that Govern Processes and Optimal Functioning.
2. State of the Art: Patterning of Human Behavior.
3. Patterning of Sleep and Respiration During Sleep.
4. Caring and Caring Lifestyles: The Central and Unifying Focus for Nursing and Doctoral Nursing Education.
5. Cooperative Program Evaluation Project in Doctoral Education in Nursing
    Part A: Introduction, Methods, Characteristics of Programs, Students, Alumni, Faculty.
    Part B: Study Findings and Plans for the Future.
6. Educational Testing Service.

In 1981, the tone of the conference shifted to *outcomes focus and research productivity*. Competing theories of science (alternative theories of science and alternative theories of theory) were detailed. Changes in philosophy of science and the views of Thomas S. Kuhn were presented along with discussion on the concept of "paradigm." The advantages and disadvantages of mentorship were analyzed. Mentorship as essential to scholarship and profiles of effective mentors were detailed. Discussion also took place on funding availability for doctoral programs and for research. The final report of the cooperative evaluation project on doctoral education in nursing was distributed (Proceedings of the 1981 Forum on Doctoral Education in Nursing).

Place: University of Washington School of Nursing
Date: June 25–26, 1981
Topics:
  1. Competing Theories of Science.
  2. Mentorship for Scholarliness.
  3. Mentorship for Scholarship: A Con Position.
  4. Programmatic Structures for Research Productivity.
  5. Structures for Research Productivity.

Substantive content in doctoral education in nursing was the essence of the 1982 national forum. Helen Grace's keynote address focused on building nursing knowledge and the current state of doctoral education. At this point in time, 23 doctoral programs were in existence. The continued need for doctoral education in nursing was detailed, with doctoral preparation in "nursing education" as the major focus. A nursing research analysis noted a true shift and increasing trend toward clinical investigation as well. Sociocultural content, the biophysiological domain, and psychosocial aspects of doctoral education were also topics of discussion (Proceedings of the 1982 Forum on Doctoral Education in Nursing).

Place: Case Western Reserve University
Date: June 24–25, 1982
Topics:
1. Substantive Content in the Sociocultural Domain.
2. Substantive Content in the Biophysiological Domain.
3. Substantive Content in the Psychosocial Domain.
4. Integration of the Domains.
5. An Integrated Biopsychosocial View of Knowledge Related to Health and Nursing.

In 1983, nurse leaders met at NYU to examine the *content of current nursing dissertations to describe substantive content*. Loomis indicated that almost 80 percent of dissertations reviewed from 1976–1982 were clinical in scope with the remainder addressing social issues in nursing. Analyzing dissertation content by type of degree—PhD, DNS, and EdD—Loomis also found significant differences. Student views, as expressed by a nationwide survey of doctoral nurses, were stressed. Discussion on nursing research grants and doctoral study for part-time students concluded the conference (Proceedings of the 1983 Forum on Doctoral Education in Nursing).

Place: New York University Division of Nursing
Date: June 23–24, 1983
Topics:
1. Substantive Content in Nursing: An Analysis of Dissertation Abstracts and Titles (1976–1982).
2. Substantive Content in Nursing: The Students' View as Expressed in a Nationwide Survey.
3. Discussion of Nursing Research Emphasis Grants.
4. Part-time Doctoral Students: Needs and Strengths.

The 1984 forum focused mainly on *philosophies and distinctions in education, research, and practice* in (clinical) doctoral programs. Clearly, unrest on the strengths and differences between doctoral degree types was evident. With two-track doctoral programs developing, concern was expressed. Quality dimensions and control, and post-doctoral training, were also debated. A study of trends and patterns of student research from 1981–1984 reflected programmatic goals (Proceedings of the 1984 Forum on Doctoral Education in Nursing).

Place: University of Colorado School of Nursing
Date: June 21–22, 1984
Topics:
1. The Research Doctorate.
2. The Doctor of Nursing Science at The Catholic University of America.
3. Textual Analysis of Doctoral Nursing Dissertation Abstracts.
4. Operationalization of Quality Dimensions in Nursing Doctoral Programs.
5. What Characterizes Quality Control in Doctoral Programs?
6. Postdoctoral Training for Research Program Development.
7. Nursing Knowledge Development.
8. The Research Doctorate (PhD) and the Professional Doctorate (DNS).
9. The Clinical Doctorate

The 1985 forum focused on *health* related to knowledge development, critical social theory, and factors influencing healthy doctoral programs. Feminist theory was also emphasized for knowledge development, although, at this time, nursing literature on theory and knowledge development made no reference to feminist theory. Nonetheless, examining knowing and feminist perspective would impact on nursing research and the development of nursing knowledge. Further emphasized was the significance of women's health and family health. Another important issue was assessment of quality in doctoral programs. The most significant standard for assessing the quality of a doctoral program involved the scholarship of the faculty as measured by publications, funding, rank, and involvement in professional activities. Other factors included quality of teaching, concern for students, resources, and students' satisfaction (Proceedings of the 1985 Forum on Doctoral Education in Nursing).

Place: University of Alabama School of Nursing
Date: June 13–14, 1985
Topics:
1. Health as Expanding Consciousness.
2. Nursing Knowledge Development: What is Health?
3. Toward a Theory of Family Health.
4. Critical Social Theory: Philosophical and Historical Dimensions of Health.
5. The Idea of Health.
6. Health: From Concept to Empirical Dimensions.
7. Healthy Doctoral Programs: The Effect of the Environment of the Nursing Doctoral Programs on Faculty and Alumni Productivity.
8. What is a Healthy Doctoral Program?
9. An Administrator's Perspective.
10. A Faculty Member's Perspective.
11. A Doctoral Student's Perspective.

Nineteen eighty-six marked the turn of a decade with the tenth national forum on doctoral education in nursing; 33 doctoral programs were in existence. *Person/Environment Interaction* provided a theme with historical, philosophical, and conceptual aspects. Central issues related to the provision of creative educational environments in doctoral programs were discussed and the announcement of the start of the National Center for Nursing Research was made. Round table discussions were held addressing such topics as funding, course work, recruitment and admission, meeting student needs, program evaluation, and post-doctoral education (Proceedings of the 1986 Forum on Doctoral Education in Nursing).

Place: University of California School of Nursing
Date: June 11–13, 1986
Topics:
1. Historical Perspective on Client/Environment Interaction.
2. Client/Environment Interaction: An Epistemological Approach.
3. Individual/Environment Transactions: Synergy and Specificity Underlying Human Response.
4. Client/Environment Interaction: Theoretical and Conceptual Perspectives about Nursing Technology.
5. Feminism, Knowledge Development, and Client/Environment Interaction.
6. Person and World: A Philosophical/Ontological Perspective.
7. Methodological Issues: The Person in Person/Environment Nursing Research.
8. A Contextual Analysis of Faculty Productivity.
9. Student Support: Relationship to Quality Indicators.
10. Environment/Person in Doctoral Programs: Faculty/Student Interaction.
11. Dimensions of the Scholarly Environment: Context for Creativity.

Since the inception of the national forums on doctoral education one sees a shift in terms of relevant issues and concerns of nursing leaders involved in the development of these programs. For example, at the inception, curricula and resources were of concern, moving to knowledge issues and substantive content in nursing. The central focus of the 1987 conference was related to *policy issues.* Concerns voiced by speakers at this conference included discussion of issues related to the intent of doctoral education, utilization of faculty with non-nursing doctorates, faculty preparation for non-research institutions, and issues surrounding quality control.

Research as a strategy for influencing practice and environmental health policy was also emphasized along with strategies for influencing public policy. Strategies and implementation of public policy related to knowledge development, education, and community mental health were further addressed. Issues and concerns related to post-doctoral education, funding opportunities, program and networking issues, diversity, and quality indicators for new doctoral programs became prominent (Proceedings of the 1987 Annual Forum on Doctoral Education in Nursing).

Place: The University of Pittsburgh School of Nursing
Date: June 25–26, 1987
Topics:
1. History as a Strategy for Shaping Educational Policy.
2. Research as a Strategy for Influencing Health Policy.
3. Futurism as a Strategy for Shaping Social Welfare Policy.
4. Strategies for Shaping Public Policy: Social Welfare.
5. Implementing Strategies for Shaping Public Policy: Physiology.
6. Implementing Strategies for Shaping Public Policy: Education.
7. Implementing Strategies for Shaping Public Policy: Community Mental Health.
8. Toward the Future.

The 1988 forum focused on *history and philosophy of science* as they related to doctoral nursing education. Position papers addressed issues in the philosophy of science in the life of an educated person.

History and feminist critique were also addressed within the context of nursing science development. Another valuable area involved history and philosophical influences on biological science development and the need for a multimethod, multidisciplinary approach to nursing science development. Educators participating in the conference were encouraged to think creatively and broadly in generating viable curriculum models to include the historical and philosophical background needed by doctoral students (Proceedings of the 1988 Forum on Doctoral Education in Nursing).

Place: University of Arizona College of Nursing
Date: June 15–17, 1988
Topics:
Position Papers
1. Role of History and Philosophy of Science in the Life of an Educated Person.
2. History and Philosophy of Science: Implications in Nursing and Biological Sciences.
3. History and Philosophy of Science: Its Implications in Nursing and Social Science.
4. Philosophy of Nursing and Nursing Science: Impact on Nursing Research.
5. *Challenge Paper*—Models for Implementing Ethics, History, and Philosophy of Science in Doctoral Curricula.

The thirteenth national forum on doctoral education in nursing focused on *where we are in the development of knowledge for doctoral programs in nursing*. Papers presented concerned one of three common conceptual bases for the organization and advancement of nursing knowledge: clinical content, nursing's metaparadigm domain concepts, and nursing diagnosis and taxonomy. Future directions for substantive knowledge development, alternative research methods, and future areas in need of knowledge development in nursing were also discussed (Proceedings of the 1989 Forum on Doctoral Education in Nursing).

Place: Indiana University School of Nursing
Date: June 7–9, 1989
Topics:
Position Papers
1. Conceptual Bases for the Organization and Advancement of Nursing Knowledge: Clinical Content.
2. A Conceptual Base for the Organization and Advancement of Nursing Knowledge: Nursing's Metaparadigm Domain Concepts.
3. Conceptual Basis for the Organization and Advancement of Nursing Knowledge: Nursing Diagnosis/Taxonomy.
4. *Challenge Paper*—Future Directions for Substantive Knowledge from Passion for Substance to *Informed* Passion. Human Science: Human Caring.

In 1990, the forum considered *alternative approaches to organizing and advancing nursing knowledge*. Alternative intellectual approaches from a variety of ways of knowing and how nurse scholars are prepared in their individual programs and research backgrounds were emphasized. Preparation of individuals capable of developing research careers dedicated to the investigation of clinical phenomenon was another topic of concern. Some attendees challenged the idea of multiple approaches to nursing research and advocated a single paradigm to build nursing knowledge. The advancement of nursing knowledge was clearly the focus and issues surrounding what type of program would best prepare nurse scholars emerged. The two degree types addressed were the PhD degree (whose major purpose traditionally is directed toward the preparation of scholars who generate new knowledge for the discipline) and the practice-oriented degrees, such as the DSN, DNS, and DNSc (Proceedings of the 1990 Forum on Doctoral Education in Nursing).

Place: University of Texas
Date: 1990
Topics:
1. Preparation of Nursing Scholars.
2. Preparation of Nursing Scholars: Alternative Approaches to Organizing and Advancing Nursing Knowledge.
3. Preparation of Nursing Scholars: Alternative Approaches to Organizing and Advancing Nursing Knowledge.
4. Conceptualizations of Nursing: Alternative Approaches to Preparing Nurse Scholars "Substance, Syntax, and Science."
5. Alternative Approaches to Preparing Nursing Scholars: Issues Concerning Uniformity and Diversity in Doctoral Programs.
6. Challenge Address: Human Neuroplasticity: Potential for Change.

Round Table Discussions:
7. Admissions, Progression, Retention.
8. Clinical Specialization.
9. Educational Funding Opportunities.
10. Methods and Tools in Research.
11. Nursing Informatics.
12. Post-doctoral Education.
13. Quality Indicators of Dissertations.
14. Socialization of Doctoral Faculty.
15. Socialization of Doctoral Faculty to New Doctoral Programs.
16. Socialization of Doctoral Students.

The 1991 meeting proposed *post-doctoral education for nursing* as its central theme. Initially explored was the progress made by institutions preparing doctoral students toward a lifetime of research. An added effort here involved understanding how nursing might grow in post-doctoral research via the basic and behavioral sciences. Federal imperatives for funding research were another topic along with indicators of quality in a post-doctoral proposal. Factors influencing the post-doctoral research experience were related to the mentor's role, funding, the purpose of post-doctoral education for clinical practice, research, and leadership in nursing (Proceedings of the 1991 Forum on Doctoral Education in Nursing).

Place: Amelia Island Plantation
Date: June 2–4, 1991
Topics:
   1. Post-doctoral Education in the Basic Sciences.
   2. Some Observations on the Nature of and Access to Post-doctoral Training in the Behavioral Sciences.
   3. Reflections on Post-graduate Studies in Nursing.
   4. The Federal Imperative in Funding Post-doctoral Education.
   5. The Minor in Doctoral Education: Relationship to Post-doctoral Research.
   6. Prevailing Paradigms in Nursing.
   7. Division of Nursing Update.
   8. Selected Health Care Data.

The 1992 forum on doctoral nursing education addressed issues surrounding *nursing as a human science*. A pluralistic, multidimensional, multi-paradigm approach alongside middle range theories crucial for guiding research and practice were encouraged. Federal updates from the National Center for Nursing Research were discussed. In addition, issues for doctoral education surrounding academic and scientific misconduct were explored (Proceedings of the 1992 Forum on Doctoral Education in Nursing).

Place: University of Maryland School of Nursing
Date: June 3–5, 1992
Topics:
   1. From Truth to Relativism: Paradigms for Doctoral Education.

(*continued*)
2. Paradigms, Socialization and Nursing Science.
3. Implications of the Particulate-Deterministic Paradigm.
4. Implications of the Interactive-Integrative Paradigm.
5. Implications of the Unitary-Transformative Paradigm.
6. Implications of the Feminist/Critical Theory Perspective.
7. Academic and Scientific Misconduct: Issues for Doctoral Nursing Education.

In 1993, *a call for substance, preparing leaders for global health,* prevailed. Participants focused on global health care issues and the unique role nurses can play in improving health for all. The substantive basis of nursing, with its varying perspectives, continued to stimulate dialogue. The National Center for Nursing Research reviewed research goals and priorities. Legislative changes and financial support that affect monies for doctoral programs were also addressed (Proceedings of the 1993 Forum on Doctoral Education in Nursing).

Place: University of Minnesota School of Nursing
Date: June 3–5, 1993
Topics:
1. A Passion for Substance Revisited: Global Transitions and International Commitments.
2. Critical Phenomena of Nursing Science: Age is Not (Just) a Demographic Variable.
3. A Substantive Focus for Nursing Science.
4. Identifying the Critical Phenomena of Nursing as Nursing Itself—Innate Developmental Processes of Health.
5. Response to the Critical Phenomena of Nursing Papers.
6. Critique of Critical Phenomena of Nursing Science, suggested by O'Brien, Reed, and Stevenson.
7. Critique: Focus on Therapeutics

(*continued*)
8. A Global Road Less Travelled: The Challenge of
Critical Phenomena in Nursing Knowledge.

In 1994 the forum dealt with visions of nursing in the twenty-first century. Perspectives on doctoral education from individuals in the programs: their roles, educational models, and the contexts in which such models were enacted were discussion topics. Additional dialogue on personal characteristics for graduates to possess, nature of role, and the nature of knowledge that should be emphasized in doctoral programs generated much interest (Proceedings of the 1994 Forum on Doctoral Education in Nursing).

Place: University of Utah
Date: June 1–3, 1994
Topics:
1. Re-Invigoration of Doctoral Education in Nursing: The Substance of Community Health and the Ethic of Partisan Alliance with Vulnerable Populations.
2. Developing a National Nursing Community While Celebrating Diversity.
3. Breakout Sessions: Doctoral Program Core Content, Substance Versus Process in Doctoral Education, Core Curriculum for Doctoral Education, Curriculum.

Since the inception of the Doctoral Education in Nursing Forums, concern about differences in the degrees offered as well as concern about the nature of nursing science, quality control, and the development and advancement of nursing knowledge has emerged. Most recently, focus has been on post-doctoral research and the development of a lifetime of scholarly work for nurses prepared at the doctoral level. The theme and focus of the forum are mandated by participants of the previous years and forums are anticipated and planned for as far into the future as the year 2004. The entire collection of *Forum Proceedings* (1977 to 1995) to date are available for reference to members and nurse scholars at the Sigma Theta Tau International Center for Nursing Scholarship Library and Information Center. The forums are important, not only for the exchange and generation of new ideas, but also in tracking trends and development of doctoral education in nursing.

SUMMARY

Doctoral education in nursing has evolved dramatically since its initial introduction as a terminal degree in nursing. The leadership provided by those nurses prepared in departments of education and other related disciplines led the way for the development of doctorates in and of nursing. Today's leaders in nursing continue to refine and evaluate the process of doctoral education in nursing through publication and the annual forums on doctoral education in nursing. As we move toward the twenty-first century, nursing clearly has developed the leadership, substantive knowledge, and direction for ensuring the preparation of future nursing leaders.

Anecdotes Reflecting Early Doctoral
Preparation For Nurses

The following quotes represent the voices of doctoral graduates whose educational experiences have varied across time and curriculums:

> I completed my doctoral program in the 1950s. My degree, the PhD, was in the Division of Social Sciences at the University of Chicago. My major was Administration in Higher Education.

> I was among the first 100 RNs to obtain a doctoral degree of any kind. This, I believe, impacted the quality and characteristics of doctoral degree programs for nurses in that era.

I haven't found doctorates to be outstanding practitioners; having knowledge, yes, professional, yes, learners, yes—but poor on giving patient care—some feel they are "above that."

I earned my doctorate over 20 years ago when the research emphasis was "simpler." There was minimal attention to philosophy of science and theories.

It was during 1949–1953. Nurse faculty didn't know much about university education and research. The *Journal of Nursing Research* appeared in 1952. Qualitative research was virtually unknown. Doctoral students didn't get together and many were part time. Full time scholarship, supporting PhD study for qualified nurses should be a major aim.

I did my doctorate at Harvard University Graduate School of Education and was the first nurse to go through their doctoral program. If one was registered in any one school one was free to take courses in any other school—hence the flexibility. I made out my own curriculum plan, it was approved by my advisor, and I moved at my own rate. Teachers were challenging and stimulating. It was the best educational experience I had ever had.

Since my education beyond my RN (1942) was partly in nursing education: MA, Teachers College Columbia University (1947) and Chemistry MA at Columbia University in 1947; and my doctoral studies were in the department of Biochemistry, the School of Hygiene and Public Health of Johns Hopkins University in 1949, my answers seem irrelevant (this reference is to the visual analog scale which comprised the quantitative aspect of this study). In those days there were very few doctoral programs for nurses. Also in those days there was not general acceptance of nurses pursuing graduate studies.

References

American Nurses' Foundation. (1969). Directory of nurses with earned doctoral degrees. *Nursing Research, 18,* 465–480.

Berelson, B. (1960). *Graduate education in the United States.* New York: McGraw-Hill.

Doctoral Education in Nursing Forum. (1977). *Proceedings of the 1977*

Forum on Doctoral Education in Nursing. Philadelphia: University of Pennsylvania.

Doctoral Education in Nursing Forum. (1978). *Proceedings of the 1978 Forum on Doctoral Education in Nursing.* Chicago: Rush University.

Doctoral Education in Nursing Forum. (1979). *Proceedings of the 1979 Forum on Doctoral Education in Nursing.* San Francisco: University of California.

Doctoral Education in Nursing Forum. (1980). *Proceedings of the 1980 Forum on Doctoral Education in Nursing.* Detroit: Wayne State University.

Doctoral Education in Nursing Forum. (1981). *Proceedings of the 1981 Forum on Doctoral Education in Nursing.* Seattle: University of Washington.

Doctoral Education in Nursing Forum. (1982). *Proceedings of the 1982 Forum on Doctoral Education in Nursing.* Cleveland: Case Western Reserve University.

Doctoral Education in Nursing Forum. (1983). *Proceedings of the 1983 Forum on Doctoral Education in Nursing.* New York: New York University.

Doctoral Education in Nursing Forum. (1984). *Proceedings of the 1984 Forum on Doctoral Education in Nursing.* Denver: University of Colorado.

Doctoral Education in Nursing Forum (1985). *Proceedings of the 1985 Forum on Doctoral Education in Nursing.* Birmingham: University of Alabama.

Doctoral Education in Nursing Forum (1986). *Proceedings of the 1986 Forum on Doctoral Education in Nursing.* San Francisco: University of California.

Doctoral Education in Nursing Forum (1987). *Proceedings of the 1987 Forum on Doctoral Education in Nursing.* Pittsburgh: University of Pittsburgh.

Doctoral Education in Nursing Forum (1988). *Proceedings of the 1988 Forum on Doctoral Education in Nursing.* Tucson: University of Arizona College of Nursing.

Doctoral Education in Nursing Forum (1989). *Proceedings of the 1989 Forum on Doctoral Education in Nursing.* Indianapolis: Indiana University School of Nursing.

Doctoral Education in Nursing Forum (1990). *Proceedings of the 1990 Forum on Doctoral Education in Nursing.* Austin: The University of Texas at Austin School of Nursing.

Doctoral Education in Nursing Forum (1991). *Proceedings of the 1991 Forum on Doctoral Education in Nursing.* Amelia Island, FL: University of Florida.

Doctoral Education in Nursing Forum (1992). *Proceedings of the 1992 Forum on Doctoral Education in Nursing.* Baltimore: University of Maryland at Baltimore.

Doctoral Education in Nursing Forum (1993). *Proceedings of the 1993 Forum on Doctoral Education in Nursing.* Saint Paul: University of Minnesota.

Doctoral Education in Nursing Forum (1994). *Proceedings of the 1994 Forum on Doctoral Education in Nursing.* Park City: The University of Utah.

Elkins, W. (1960). Doctoral education in nursing—A university president presents his point of view. *Nursing Outlook, 35,* 136–140.

Gorney-Fadiman, M. (1981). A student's perspective on the doctoral dilemma. *Nursing Outlook, 29,* 650–654.

Grace, H. K. (1978). The development of doctoral education in nursing: In historical perspective. *Journal of Nursing Education, 17,* 17–29.

Grace, H. K. (1989). Issues in Doctoral Education in Nursing. *Journal of Professional Nursing, 5*(5), 266–270.

Hassenplug, L. (1966). Doctoral preparation for nurses—A continuation of the dialogue. *Nursing Forum, 5,* 53–56.

Leininger, M. (1974). Scholars, scholarship, and nursing scholarship. *Image, 6*(2), 5–14.

Malden, H. (1835). *On the origin of universities and academic degrees.* London: John Taylor.

Marriner-Tomey, A. (1990). Historical development of doctoral programs from the middle ages to nursing education today. *Nursing & Health Care, 11*(3), 133–137.

Matarazzo, J., & Abdellah, F. (1971). Doctoral education for nursing in the United States. *Nursing Research, 33,* 139–143.

McManus, L. (1960). Doctoral education in nursing—a nurse educator responds. *Nursing Outlook, 8*(10), 543–545.

Murphy, J. F. (1981). Doctoral education in, of, and for nursing: An historical analysis. *Nursing Outlook, 29,* 645–649.

Newman, M. (1975). The professional doctorate in nursing: Position paper. *Nursing Outlook, 23,* 704–706.

Nichols, R. F. (1967). A reconsideration of the PhD. *The Graduate School, 7,* 327–328.

Parietti, E. S. (1979). *Development of doctoral education for nurses: An historical survey.* Unpublished doctoral dissertation, Teachers College, Columbia University.

Spurr, S. H. (1970). *Academic degree structures: Innovative approaches.* New York: McGraw-Hill.

Veysey, L. (1973). *Stability and experiment in the American undergraduate curriculum.* New York: McGraw-Hill.

Werley, H., & Leske, J. (1988). Pinning down the tracks to doctoral degrees. *Nursing and Health Care, 9,* 239–243.

CHAPTER TWO

On Program Choice

No doctoral program prepares an excellent researcher, administrator, or practitioner. Excellence (expertise) comes only with years of practice and years of research on the same topic and with the same method and with publication of results.

Diversity it is said, lends strength to a discipline. As for variation in doctoral degrees in nursing, the answer is yes.

Students' Comments

INTRODUCTION

IN 1989, FLORENCE DOWNS WROTE:

When I began to think about preparing this article, it struck me that my educational history had come home to roost. When I entered New York University many years ago as a post-baccalaureate student, something virtually unheard of in nursing at that time, I matriculated on an EdD. Later, I was persuaded to rematriculate for a PhD. Still later, I was persuaded to rematriculate again for an EdD. By the time I completed my dissertation, I had met the requirements for both degrees, 105 credits beyond the baccalaureate. At the final oral examination, a reader asked on what degree I was matriculated. When I said I believed it was the EdD, the reader responded, "but this is a PhD dissertation." I told him I was unaware there was a difference between a PhD and an EdD dissertation. If I had known then that I would be standing here discussing differences between the DNS and the PhD, I certainly would have asked what distinguished the EdD from the PhD. Perhaps it would not have helped, because educators still indulge in debates about the differences that have surrounded doctoral education since it was introduced in this country (Downs, 1989, p. 261).

The words of Florence Downs are still echoed by many doctoral students today and a review of curriculums in doctoral nursing programs reveals a similar situation. Although we talk about theoretical differences, such as, the EdD being the pedagogical degree; the DNS being the professional degree; and the PhD being the research degree; in fact, doctoral students perceive very little difference between the three types of programs. Further, the published literature suggests that differences among program type are almost impossible to discern, with research being the primary emphasis whether the degree is the EdD, PhD, or DNS.

Discussions of the nature, similarities, and differences between programs for earning a doctorate are not uncommon and models for doctoral education in nursing continue to be examined. Recognizing that the requirements of a practice discipline are very different from academic disciplines, nursing has viewed all possible higher education models in an attempt to identify the most appropriate direction for doctoral education in nursing. Recently, the trend has been toward development of the PhD in nursing rather than the DNS, a pattern that moves the profession away from its practice base and closer to an academic model. Faculty practice is still required, however, if nursing plans to continue to recruit and educate both new and advanced practice nurses. This requirement is more congruent with the professional model. This chapter reviews the types of doctoral programs in nursing available to nurses pursuing advanced education. A discussion of student perceptions regarding similarities and differences among the program types is included.

DOCTORATES IN NURSING: AN OVERVIEW OF THE LITERATURE

Doctoral preparation as an educational pathway for nurses has evolved dramatically since its inception in the 1920s. The 59 doctoral nursing programs educating nurses today offer a variety of doctoral degrees, and include the PhD, EdD, DNS (or DNSc) and Nurse Doctorate (ND) programs. Several doctoral nursing programs offer two degree types such as the PhD or the DNS.

Prospective students have a variety of doctoral program choices and may select a particular program based on both academic and personal need. One very important issue in doctoral nursing education is whether the diversity in degrees that exists is needed in the profession. Ziemer (1992) noted that the growing trend is toward emphasis on the PhD, or what is considered by some to be the academic research doctorate. This trend has been supported in the literature (Andreoli, 1986; Brown, 1985; Forni, 1989; Meleis, 1988; Rogers, 1966).

Diversity has been recommended and viewed positively by others as well (Booth, 1989; Downs, 1988; Moccia, 1986). Starck, Duffy, and Vogler (1993) suggested that an "expert practitioner" with a "concentrated focus on the acquisition of high-level scientific knowledge" (p. 213) is needed; that is, a practice-based doctorate or DNS degree.

In contemporary nursing literature, analysis of the varying nursing doctorates is offered by several authors (Anderson, Roth & Palmer, 1985; Anderson, 1989; Brodie, 1986; Blancett, 1989; Barnum, 1991; Casserett, 1989; Seitz, 1987). It is generally agreed upon by nurse doctorates that the EdD tends to be a pedagogical degree; the PhD a research or academic degree; and the DNS the clinical research degree.

The broad requirements of nursing and non-nursing programs focus on mastery of a specific body of knowledge, research and competence, as well as the design and completion of research in one's area of specialization (Harris, Trout & Andrews, 1980; Pitel & Vian, 1975). Program requirements in doctoral nursing education remain consistent with those of other professions. Most offer the student advanced nursing theory, qualitative and quantitative research methodologies, and assistance in completion and publication of nursing research. Beare, Gray and Ptak (1981) studied PhD and EdD doctoral programs and noted that all programs included nursing theory, theory development, concept formulation and quantitative analysis.

Snyder-Halpern (1986) studied four PhD and DNS programs in order to evaluate curricular design and outcome variables. Close similarities were found in curricular content in PhD and DNS programs. Both programs geared students toward roles as educators and applied researchers. One difference was in clinical preparation. The DNS programs prepared clinicians and the PhD programs prepared students more oriented to research. Both Meleis (1988) and Gorney-Fadiman (1981) noted similar viewpoints.

Curran, Habeeb, and Sobol (1981) discussed the dilemma of selecting a doctoral program for a nursing career due to the variety of program types. The authors noted that differences in programs are just not clear. "A persistent myth identifies the DNS as a practice degree; however, the DNS does not propose to prepare clinical practitioners" (p. 37). According to the authors, degrees such as the PhD or EdD are well established in academic communities—the DNS is not.

Downs (1989) reviewed curricular requirements in 43 DNS and PhD programs. She found that DNS programs had considerably more clinical hours documented whereas PhD programs placed more emphasis on statistics and research.

Farren (1991) suggested that degree type influences research activity. In a study of 152 nurses with doctorates, degree type was significantly related to research productivity. Nurses with PhDs and those with DNS degrees were found to be the top research producing groups, while the same study reported that nurse doctorates (NDs) were less likely to conduct research. Ninety-six percent of all those studied, however, felt competent to actually perform research investigations.

A recent study conducted by Ziemer and colleagues (1992) examined the philosophy, curricula, and program requirements of 44 doctoral nursing programs. The following types of programs were analyzed in this study: EdD, PhD and DNS. Similarities were noted among program types with consistent emphasis on clinical or role development and research preparation. Ketefian (1993) emphasized the need to focus on nursing content rather than on process courses in doctoral curricula (i.e., research, history of nursing and statistics).

Dennis (1991) emphasized the need for doctoral preparation to facilitate the role of clinical nurse researcher.

Other issues affecting this level of education include program quality, academic rigor, and the ability to perform and publish research. Program quality is also a concern due to the rapid proliferation of doctoral programs. The lack of faculty with adequate research backgrounds and productivity relates to this issue (Anderson, 1989).

Several authors (Andreoli, 1986; Brimmer, 1983; Sherwin, Bevil, Adler & Watson, 1993) have addressed the continued need for nurses with doctorates. Additionally, doctorally prepared faculty will be needed to ensure health care security (Ketefian, 1993). For an extensive review of the literature on doctoral education the reader is referred to Hudacek and Carpenter (1994).

Grace (1978) and Murphy (1981) traced the historical development of doctoral education for nurses and considered the development in three steps: 1) Doctoral education for nurses in education and administration; 2) Doctoral education for nurses in a discipline other than nursing; and 3) Doctoral education for nurses, in the discipline of nursing. Stevenson and Woods (1986) gave a four-step description of doctoral education in nursing that correlates closely with trends noted in the *Annual Forums on Doctoral Education in Nursing,* reviewed in Chapter 1.

Stevenson and Woods (1986) noted that from 1900 through 1940, the first generation consisted of nurses with the EdD or other functional doctorates. The second generation (1940–1960) earned PhDs in the basic or social sciences with no nursing content. The third generation, in the 1960s, included the PhDs in basic sciences with a minor in nursing. The fourth and present generation (1970–present) is that of the doctorate in nursing, PhD, or doctorate of nursing science (DNS). The next generation (2000 and beyond) is projected to be one of "greater specificity within nursing" and "formalized postdoctoral programs" (Stevenson & Woods, 1986, p. 8).

The discussion that follows addresses each type of doctorate currently offered in nursing, including the EdD, DNS (or DNSc), PhD, and ND degree.

THE DOCTOR OF EDUCATION IN NURSING (EdD)

When doctoral education in nursing began, programs were primarily located in schools of education. Nurses initially prepared at the doctoral level attended well established programs in education. Teachers College at Columbia University and the School of Education at New York University were preparing the majority of these nurses. Discussions about whether nursing is a practice discipline, a clinical science, or a basic science began in these early programs (Downs, 1989).

The first program offering a doctorate for nurses in the early 1900s was at Teachers College, and nurses there participated in areas of study and research most relevant to their practice. At that time, for most of these nursing leaders, practice meant teaching and managing as opposed to clinical nursing practice. These early nursing leaders were educators and administrators earning doctoral preparation congruent with their work and careers. According to Baer (1987), the competition among nursing's teaching, managing, and practice roles, present from nursing's American origins, found its expression in research conducted at the time. In other words, research conducted by these early nursing leaders did not stem from a clinical practice base or the substantive knowledge of nursing. Rather, these early nursing leaders conducted research related to their educational and administrative roles.

Teachers College continues to prepare nurses at the doctoral level today, and nurses studying for the doctorate in this program are earning the EdD in nursing. Curriculum requirements have changed with the times, and the program at Teachers College has evolved to match the expectations of the profession. This program continues to offer the only EdD in nursing.

Narrative comments from participants of the study reported on in this book view the EdD in Nursing as the degree that prepares students for positions in education, as well as a degree that prepares students to conduct research in their area of interest. Doctoral work which results in the awarding of the EdD degree is viewed as preparation for those individuals wishing to become faculty and curriculum leaders. Some participants believed that nurses should no longer participate in EdD education and that all doctoral preparation should have as its ultimate goal, the earning of the PhD. This was related to the fact that the PhD is viewed as being more credible outside of nursing, and more accepted among academic disciplines. Students continue to earn the EdD in nursing, and make their choice based on a clear knowledge of their personal career goals and needs. According to one participant:

> It took me over ten years post-Masters to decide on the doctoral program of my choice. Some of the factors that contributed to the length between graduate programs are directly related to the profession's bickering and condescension over the worthiness of various degrees. It was only after Lucy Kelly's editorial in *Nursing Outlook* (I think it was Lucy Kelly) that called for an end to this in-house squabble, along with the Carnegie Report on Scholarship Revisited, that I engaged in the educational process that will hopefully result in the EdD. The EdD is the doctoral degree I have always wanted to pursue—Why?—Because it fits my philosophical beliefs about who and what I am as a professional and as a nurse educator.

THE DOCTOR OF NURSING SCIENCE (DNS)

The DNS program of study was developed to emphasize advanced clinical practice. Integrating research and practice with the development of nursing knowledge and the improvement of nursing practice were central to this program's development. Although many DNS programs are located in health science centers, it is common knowledge that in some instances the professional doctorate was chosen because the institution offered no mechanism for establishing the PhD. The DNS degree was developed for a variety of reasons including the fit with the school's resources and the consideration of university resources in support of the program (Forni & Welch, 1987).

Newman noted in 1975 that nursing was having difficulty demonstrating its value to the public, a problem that continues to plague the profession today. She suggested that the professional doctorate was one mechanism for nursing to have equal status with other major health professionals. Newman (1975) further noted that the professional doctorate is similar to the Doctor of Medicine degree, a practice doctorate that constitutes basic preparation for practice.

The professional doctorate in nursing is generally construed to be the practice-oriented, clinical or applied degree and implies preparation for a practice role of some sort. These roles may be administrator, teacher, or clinical researcher. The professional model results in a practice-focused degree that is based upon a baccalaureate foundation (Forni & Welch, 1987). According to Forni and Welch (1987), "It is well recognized that currently some programs that offer the DNS degree are more like PhD programs in their academic requirements and vice versa" (p. 294).

The literature abounds with discussions about the DNS, and the importance of preparing doctoral candidates that are grounded in practice. Christman (1978) stated this concern very clearly:

> If nursing is to be fully accepted as a profession, it will require a complete educational system that will enable nurses to achieve excellence in service, education, and research. Educational preparation for this kind of leadership must be anchored solidly in the central concern of nurses—the clinical nursing care of patients (Christman, 1978, p. 45).

THE DOCTOR OF PHILOSOPHY DEGREE (PhD)

The PhD emphasizes the development and advancement of nursing knowledge. The policy statement of the Association of Graduate Schools identifies the PhD as the highest achievement in preparation for active scholarship and research, noting that the nature and purpose of the PhD is to: (1) prepare students for a lifetime of intellectual inquiry, creative scholarship and research; (2) lead to careers in government, business, and industry, as well as academia; and (3) result in extension of knowledge (The Council of Graduate

Schools, 1977, p. 1). The trend toward the PhD in nursing is clear, with the majority of doctoral programs in nursing offering this type of degree. Lash (1987) discussed at length the nature of the PhD and noted that "despite varying practices in labeling degrees, the PhD is associated with graduate school and advanced learning in the United States and has achieved supremacy over other doctoral degrees" (p. 92).

Narrative comments from doctoral students involved in PhD programs supported this track for nursing. Rationale for the PhD as perceived by students enrolled in these programs was related to beliefs about research preparation and credibility of the degree in other disciplines outside of nursing. Further, as students noted that their colleagues in nursing valued the PhD above other degrees, they therefore chose this avenue for their own doctoral pursuits. The absence of a clinical focus is viewed by some as a major omission in PhD programs and there is a sense that DNS and PhD programs should combine and that there should be one degree— the PhD. Students enrolled in PhD programs perceive them as adequate preparation for engaging in research. A sampling of students revealed these responses:

> The curriculum in the PhD program prepares nurse researchers primarily.

> It seems obvious to me that the PhD is the scholarly degree in nursing.

> I want to do research, so I chose a PhD program.

> You do need a PhD to begin to be a researcher.

> The problem in nursing occurs when the various levels of doctoral education in nursing are obscured by those in nursing who feel that the EdD and DNS degrees are equivalent to the PhD.

In terms of *credibility,* students commented:

> I believe the PhD should be the only doctoral degree for nurses because nurses will have more credibility with other disciplines.

I chose the PhD over an EdD because I felt the PhD was more widely recognized by all educators and non-educators.

THE NURSE DOCTORATE (ND)

Although the qualitative data reflected in this book does not include responses from students enrolled in ND programs, it is important to address this particular program type in this chapter. This degree is very different from other nursing doctorates and makes an important contribution to the advancement of nursing practice.

The nurse doctorate was introduced by Rozella M. Schlotfeldt and began at Case Western University. The idea was a creative one, and continues to have the potential to raise nursing to a professional status not yet fully recognized. Schlotfeldt's ideas and rationale for the professional doctorate, or ND degree, are both creative and in keeping with what is expected in the medical field, where no one questions professional status.

The ND was proposed by Schlotfeldt (1978) to distinguish this level of educational accomplishment from the PhD or academic doctorate. The ND degree was designed as a form of pre-service nursing education which would reorient nursing's approach to preparing professionals toward competent, independent, accountable nursing practice. Again, the ND is a pre-service degree, differing from the PhD, which indicates completion of formal research training, and from the DNS which attests to completion of the highest level of preparation for specialization in nursing practice.

> Practice disciplines that enjoy the status of professions have concomitant responsibilities that can be fulfilled only if practitioners of the disciplines have command of a vast body of distinctive, structured knowledge which they then utilize selectively with the exercise of exquisite judgment, in making decisions that are profoundly consequential (Schlotfeldt, 1978, p. 302).

Schlotfeldt (1978) noted some of the problems currently in existence in basic nursing education programs. Basic nursing programs continue to differ remarkably in content, length, rigor, and requirements, yet all graduates are admitted to the same (RN) licensing examination. "Quite obviously, an examination which is valid for students prepared as professionals cannot also be valid for students prepared as technologists; and the converse is also true" (Schlotfeldt, 1978, p. 304). Schlotfeldt (1978) further noted:

> Despite variations, there are two characteristics that many, perhaps most, baccalaureate programs hold in common. The first is a persistent orientation toward technical, as contrasted with professional study. Whereas programs of professional study in other fields characteristically require students to master vast amounts of professional content before assuming any responsibility for care or practice, students in baccalaureate nursing programs are usually expected to learn and perform certain nursing techniques and procedures in care settings almost from the beginning of their program. This persistent propensity toward having students immediately learn "to do," prior to their learning to know the discipline in which they will eventually be "doing" indicates that baccalaureate nursing students are not yet uniformly socialized toward a truly professional orientation (Schlotfeldt, 1978, p. 308).

Schlotfeldt (1978) believed that certain goals were central to the education of nursing professionals. The mastery of subject matter had to come before practice, and control over the quality of clinical learning situations was critical.

> Students seeking admission to any program of professional study, especially those classified as the helping professions, should have capacities for mastering large quantities of knowledge, for establishing and maintaining productive and helping relationships with others, for self direction, for making discriminative judgments, for systematic inquiry, and for developing social consciousness. They should be liberally educated men and women who are gifted intellectually, willing to invest themselves in a rigorous, demanding, rewarding program of study, and committed to a sustained professional career. All should have an accurate conceptualization of the profession they have selected and its potential for service to all of mankind (Schlodtfeldt, 1978, p. 309).

The ND degree continues to be offered today, with the goals of Dr. Schlodtfeldt kept central to the programs. Several other universities also offer the ND degree including Rush University and the University of Colorado.

STUDENT PERCEPTIONS REGARDING PROGRAM TYPE

Doctoral students are less concerned with the type of program in which they are enrolled, and most concerned with the quality of the program in terms of research and role preparation. There is an overriding sense that doctoral education must be in nursing, although the contributions of doctorally prepared nurses in other disciplines must be recognized. Clearly, students must clarify their own personal and professional goals prior to choosing any doctoral program, and then select a program based on personal fit and philosophy. Doctoral students perceive that this level of academic preparation is important for all nursing functions—practice, education and administration—and that research must be a primary component of all these areas.

There is a belief that clinical expertise should occur at the master's level primarily, although students do have a sense that the preparation of expert practitioners at the doctoral level needs continued exploration and development. Anger and frustration regarding differences in degree types and perceptions regarding the valuing of certain degrees is also evident in the narrative responses of students. The following quotes from participants illustrate this:

> Now it appears that only the initials behind your name are what is important.

> The DNS, ND, PhD perpetuate the educational morass that is nursing's.

> The existence of multiple doctoral degrees in nursing leads to confusion by the public and other disciplines, threatening nursing's credibility.

Clearly, doctoral students sense the differences in program type, some experiencing the differences more than others. Having a focused sense of vision about one's own goals and career path provides the overriding direction for individuals selecting a particular type of doctoral program. The PhD dominates in number in terms of the types of doctoral programs available to nurses today, and has carried with it the prestige and recognition of all academicians. Nursing's struggle for credibility among other academics and health care professionals seems to direct the path that leads toward the doctoral degree—and that path is clearly toward the PhD in nursing.

NURSE DOCTORATE CONNECTIONS

Nursing has been hashing out what the profession believes to be important for the preparation of nursing scholars. Whether or not the differences between degrees is clear to students, however, has not been explored. The following data provide the students' perspective on differences in doctoral nursing programs. Data was collected through a mailed questionnaire which requested information about research preparation, academic rigor, quality indicators, peer and faculty preparation as a practitioner, researcher, educator and administrator. Nurses from PhD, DNS, and the only existing EdD program in nursing were surveyed. The findings of this study are important to the discussion in this chapter because they address student perceptions of the differences among the three types of doctoral programs offered in nursing. Specifically, questions guiding this investigation included:

1. Do students enrolled in PhD, DNS, and EdD programs have different research preparation?
2. Do students enrolled in PhD, DNS, and EdD programs have different role preparation?
3. Do students enrolled in PhD, DNS, and EdD programs have different experiences in terms of personal and professional growth?

4. Do students enrolled in PhD, DNS, and EdD programs have different support systems in the academic setting?

Doctoral programs listed in the Sigma Theta Tau International listing from 1991 were invited to participate. Graduates from 32 PhD programs, 7 DNS programs, 2 programs that offered both the PhD/DNS degree, and the only existing EdD program in nursing returned questionnaires. Participants included 340 PhD, 47 DNS, and 13 EdD students. The average age of participants was 42 and the mean number of years of nursing experience was 18. Participants had been enrolled in doctoral education an average of three years.

The data reported here were taken from the quantitative portion of the questionnaire. There were 401 usable surveys returned, and the statistical program for the Social Sciences (SPSS) was used for all data analysis procedures. Factor analysis was performed to identify interpretable factors for the 36 items in the questionnaire and factors extracted provided both a view of the data and an explanation of variance. Common factors were extracted using the principal components method.

Four factors were identified and included: (1) research preparation, (2) functional role preparation, (3) personal and professional development, and (4) peer support. A discussion of the results related to each factor follows and provides for the reader a sense of how students enrolled in the three program types in nursing perceive their preparation in relationship to the four factors identified. This data further clarifies the similarities and differences among the degree types in doctoral nursing education.

RESEARCH PREPARATION

Students generally agree that they have been prepared for research in their doctoral programs whether the program is a DNS, PhD, or EdD. Perceptions of students enrolled in DNS programs were significantly different, however, on the research factor than subjects in EdD and PhD programs. DNS students agreed less than PhD and

EdD students that their programs prepared them for research and that research was the primary focus of their program. Students in DNS programs did not perceive the DNS degree to focus on quantitative research. In addition, this group agreed less than EdD and PhD students that statistics courses were extremely rigorous in their doctoral programs. DNS students reported that strong faculty mentorship for research was less available and that students received less dissertation support than their EdD and PhD colleagues.

ROLE PREPARATION

When subjects were asked if the doctorate prepared them for a specific role i.e., researcher, practitioner, educator or administrator, PhD students had significantly different scores than EdD and DNS students. The PhD students did not perceive the doctorate as a degree that prepared them for roles as educators, practitioners or administrators, but as researchers. In addition, PhD students did not view EdD and DNS programs as educational pathways that prepared students to engage in research.

The results indicated that students perceive research differences in the doctoral education process. DNS students have reported that research, specifically, quantitative research, was not a primary focus of the program. In addition, faculty mentorship and dissertation support were less available to DNS students than other doctoral students who participated in this study.

PERSONAL AND PROFESSIONAL GROWTH

There were no significant differences between PhD, EdD, and DNS students in the areas of personal and professional growth. Attaining a doctorate was perceived to be enriching from both a personal as well as a professional perspective, and doctoral students agreed that doctoral programs contributed to personal and professional growth. Areas in which students reported personal improvement included cognitive, problem solving and critical thinking ability. Subjects also reported greater self confidence. Professional development, particularly scholarly writing, improved in the doctoral education process as well as overall professional confidence. Personal and professional growth are discussed further in Chapter 9.

SUPPORT

A significant difference in support was not noted among the different doctoral program types, however, most participants stressed the importance of peer support and the need to learn from other students. Strong agreement was reported on the need for networking with faculty and students. Doctoral students reported supporting each other in the educational process. See Chapter 5 for a further discussion of peer support and networking.

SUMMARY

The function of doctoral study should be to help students develop the skills they need to identify and tackle what is not known in their particular areas of interest, as well as provide the opportunity to develop a depth of understanding in the research areas they wish to explore, whether they are in a PhD, DNS or EdD program.
According to Downs (1989):

> The salient issues in doctoral education in nursing should be the nature of the scholar and the nature of the scholarship we hope to produce. A healthy peer culture of students and faculty members with diverse interest provides a natural medium for exchange of opinion on philosophical, political and policy issues, as well as a learning environment that stipulates the behaviors that characterize scholars (Downs, 1989, p. 265).

Issues related to the higher education model permeate all levels of nursing education and the higher education model which nursing chooses to follow will surely have implications for nursing's future. As Forni (1989) noted:

> Given the pluralistic nature of our society and of our education network, it seems apparent that a multiplicity of programs will continue to exist and thrive. This phenomenon will serve to enrich the educational experience of the graduates and enhance the opportunities for doctoral study in nursing. What seems apparent is that there is no perfect program for preparing nurses to become researchers, teachers, administrators, and practitioners (p. 434).

Finally, Forni (1989) recommended that we heed the words of Matarazzo (1971), who noted that, "it is probably the personal characteristics of the man (or woman), and not his academic degree per se which will help determine his degree of contribution to our vast, ever-increasing output of new scientific knowledge" (Matarazzo, 1971, p. 63).

Student Comments Regarding Similarities and Differences Among Program Types in Doctoral Education in Nursing

The following quotes represent diverse student opinion and experience of various doctoral nursing programs. They are based on questionnaire responses:

> I think it is ludicrous to require all faculty to have PhDs to teach, yet do no quality control re: a person's preparation to teach.

> I have to say that, for all my work and money, I would emerge from the program with a PhD. I can't help but believe that the differences between EdDs and PhDs are minor, but there is no doubt that the PhD is more highly respected.

> The EdD, PhD, DNSC again fragments nursing, as the multiple entry levels have in the past.

I am worried about acceptance from nursing and non-nursing disciplines since I will obtain a DNS rather than a PhD.

The combination of the PhD, EdD (in nursing only), and the DNS fully legitimizes the discipline of nursing science.

It is time to delineate what core programs are essential to all doctoral programs and what elements are unique to prepare educators, researchers, etc. The EdD, PhD, DNS *again* fragments nursing, as the multiple entry levels have in the past. What other discipline has such confusion?

I do not support the idea of attaining doctoral education outside the discipline, if one is to be a scholar in one's chosen field. In addition, the DNSc degree (although there is little difference between it and a PhD in *some* programs), does not have the same status as a PhD from the perspective of other scientific disciplines. In fact, as you may well know, some schools originated the DNS because they could not get university approval for a PhD program.

We need doctorally prepared nurses at both clinical and research levels. The PhD is not well suited for clinical practice and the DNSc does not prepare a person to engage in a program of research.

One weakness of PhD programs is that they fail to adequately prepare students to be educators. Most positions available to PhDs are in academic settings. It would be helpful to be prepared as an instructor as well as a researcher.

I think it is appropriate to have different programs emphasizing different roles—clinical, research, educator—but they could all be PhD, or they would not have to be, so what.

I completed my EdD in 1979. The emphasis was on nursing education administration. I was not well prepared in research, nor was post-doctoral research encouraged. Now, 14 years later, I feel ill prepared as I attempt to move into a Deanship, and I find my experience and background in administration is devalued.

There is too much emphasis on what the initials are after an individual's name and too little on the individual's abilities. Recognition needs to be given to individual strengths and weaknesses. We need administrators, teachers, researchers who are well grounded in nursing theory and can utilize the skills of others to complement their own skills.

It is essential that more nurses be prepared at the doctoral level. I personally feel the PhD is the degree of choice, and it should be in nursing with an emphasis solely on research to improve nursing care and patient health.

I believe that the PhD is the academic degree in nursing science. As in other sciences the PhD is the capstone scholarly degree. While most professional fields have more than one doctorate, the PhD is recognized in those areas as the most rigorous, even though attribution is given to other doctorates. I believe this should also be the case in nursing. The EdD (in nursing) and the DNS are specifically designed to prepare faculty (EdD) and practitioners (DNS). They have a statistical and a research component but the emphasis is not on research or theory development for the science of nursing. The problem in nursing occurs when the various levels of doctoral education in nursing are obscured by those in nursing who feel that EdDs and DNSs are the equivalent of the PhD. Other disciplines do not have this "in fighting" over degrees. They recognize the other degrees as to their contribution to education and practice while giving full credit to the PhD for its scholarly/research/theory building strength. The combination of the PhD, the EdD (in nursing only), and the DNSC fully legitimize the discipline of nursing science.

I do not think that diversity of doctoral programs in nursing is bad. We can follow the example of older professions by clearly identifying applied/practical/professional doctorates and traditional PhDs. I share the desire to see more nurses with doctorates in nursing, but also feel that nurses with doctorates in other disciplines have much to offer the profession.

Although I must admit that I am not extremely knowledgeable about the different doctoral programs in nursing, I do believe that doctorates should be in nursing—perhaps with strong/weak influences from other disciplines. I also prefer the PhD. I think that a total immersion in research is inappropriate for nursing. More focus should be on policy, politics and more innovative practice. However, I decided on the PhD (research) degree because I felt it would be more credible outside of nursing. Once our status is improved outside of nursing then I think the DNS would be more appropriate. After all, MDs don't need PhDs.

I see a place for non-PhD doctorates in nursing only if these degrees are appreciated for their content, and that the people possessing such degrees are used appropriately on faculties, i.e., EdD prepared people are responsible for curriculum development, DNS prepared for clinical work, and PhDs for research. There can certainly be some overlap, but totally ignoring differences in educational content leads to faculty frustration, distress and inferior programs.

I believe that PhD should be the only doctoral degree for nurses because nurses will have more credibility with other disciplines. The PhD is a standard degree, one that is well-known. The existence of multiple doctoral degrees in nursing leads to confusion by the public and other disciplines thereby threatening nursing's credibility.

I wish I had spent more time in the application process to determine the differences between programs, the PhD, DNS in particular, since I knew I wanted a research focus. The fact that colleagues where I taught valued the PhD in Nursing is the reason I chose this program.

While the doctorate is considered important, I would have developed professionally without one (research, publications, etc.) because of my own goals and commitments. The doctorate helped, but has had its limitations since it is not the degree, but what one does with it and with one's self that is valued in the real world.

Doctoral education programs are very different. The PhD, EdD, or DNSC do not guarantee a rigorous research preparation. I personally do not believe any doctoral program prepares you to be the "end all" in research. The most important part of doctoral education to me was to develop as a scholar, to learn rigorous methods of thought and analysis, and to question the status quo.

Nursing continues to create messes. We can't get entry level issues solved, let alone doctoral preparation issues. There should be one degree at the doctoral level. That degree should be the PhD with the student focusing on the area which most interests him or her: research, education, administration or practice. The EdD was an appropriate degree in the past, it is not appropriate for the future.

I feel that all programs for doctoral education are of value. The focus in my EdD program has been on developing expert skills in an area of practice be it education or administration. I don't feel that one type is better than the others. We are all prepared to do scholarly work and research in our area of interest.

There is a need for three types of doctoral degrees in nursing, however, the specific degree should determine the career path.

Being doctorally prepared is an end to the means; to me it is only just the beginning of learning more about nursing and all of its aims; practice, education, research, administration.

Once our status is improved outside of nursing then I think the DNS would be more appropriate.

Nurses with doctorates in other fields are valuable and do have contributions to make, but are not as well grounded in the discipline of nursing as are those with doctorates in nursing.

References

Anderson, C. (1989). Type and expectations of faculty. *Journal of Professional Nursing, 5,* 250–255.

Anderson, E., Roth, P., & Palmer, I. (1985). A national survey of the need for doctorally prepared nurses in academic settings and health service agencies. *Journal of Professional Nursing, 1,* 23–33.

Andreoli, K. (1986). Specialization and graduate curriculum: finding the fit. *Nursing and Health Care, 8,* 65–69.

Baer, E. (1987). A cooperative venture in pursuit of professional status: A research journal for nursing. *Nursing Research, 36,* 18–25.

Barnum, B. J. (1991). Doctoral education for the nurse executive. *Nursing and Health Care Supplement,* pub. No. 41-2365, 57–59.

Beare, P., Gray, C., & Ptak, H. (1981). Doctoral curricula in nursing. *Nursing Outlook, 29,* 311–316.

Blancett, S. S. (1989). Defining doctoral education. *Nurse Educator, 14,* 3.

Booth, R. (1989). Summary of American Association of Colleges of nursing 1989 Doctoral Conference. *Journal of Professional Nursing, 5,* 271–272.

Brimmer, P., Skoner, M., Pender, N., Williams, C., Fleming, J., & Werley, H. (1983). Nurses with doctoral degrees: Education and employment characteristics. *Research in Nursing and Health, 6,* 157–165.

Brodie, B. (1986). Impact of doctoral programs on nursing education. *Journal of Professional Nursing, 2,* 350–357.

Brown, S. A. (1985). A perspective on why nurses should earn doctorates in nursing. *Perspectives in Psychiatric Care, 1,* 16–21.

Cassarett, A. (1989). Components needed to support graduate education. *Journal of Professional Nursing, 5,* 256–260.

Christman, L. (1978). Doctoral education: A shot in the arm for the nursing profession. *Nursing Digest, 6*(2), 45–46.

Curran, C., Habeeb, M., & Sobol, E. (1981). Selecting a doctoral program for a career in nursing. *Journal of Nursing Administration, 11,* 35–40.

Dennis, K. (1991). Components of the doctoral curriculum that build success in the clinical nursing researcher role. *Journal of Professional Nursing, 7*(3), 160–165.

Downs, F. (1988). Doctoral education: Our claim to the future. *Nursing Outlook, 36,* 18–20.

Downs, F. (1989). Differences between the professional doctorate and the academic/research doctorate. *Journal of Professional Nursing, 5,* 261–265.

The Doctor of Philosophy Degree: A Policy Statement. (1977). The Council of Graduate Schools in the United States: Washington, DC.

Elkins, W. (1960). Doctoral education in nursing—a university president presents his point of view. *Nursing Outlook, 8,* 542–544.

Farren, E. (1991). Doctoral preparation and research productivity. *Nursing Outlook, 39,* 22–25.

Forni, P. (1989). Models for doctoral programs: First professional degree or terminal degree. *Nursing and Health Care, 10,* 429–434.

Forni, P. R., & Welch, M. J. (1987). The professional versus the academic model: A dilemma for nursing education. *The Journal of Professional Nursing* (September–October), 291–296.

Gorney-Fadiman, M. (1981). A student's perspective on the doctoral dilemma. *Nursing Outlook, 29,* 650–654.

Grace, H. K. (1978). Issues in doctoral education in nursing. *Journal of Professional Nursing, 5,* 266–270

Harris, J. L., Trout, W., & Andrews, G. (1980). *The American Doctorate in the context of the new patterns in higher education.* Washington, DC: The Council of Postsecondary Accreditation.

Hassenplug, L. (1966). Doctoral preparation for nurses—a continuation of the dialogue. *Nursing Forum, 5,* 53–56.

Hudacek, S., & Carpenter, D. R. (1994). Doctoral education in nursing. *Review of Research in Nursing Education,* Volume VI. New York: National League for Nursing Press, Pub. No. 19-2544.

Kemble, E. (1966). Doctoral preparation for nurses—a continuation of the dialogue. *Nursing Forum, 5,* 53–56.

Ketefian, S. (1993). Doctoral preparation for faculty roles: Expectations and realities. *Journal of Professional Nursing, 7*(2), 105–111.

Lash, A. A. (1987). The nature of the doctor of philosophy degree: Evolving conceptions. *Journal of Professional Nursing* (March–April), 92–100.

Matarazzo, J. (1971). Doctoral Education for Nursing in the United States. *Nursing Research, 33,* 139–143.

McManus, L. (1960). Doctoral education nursing—a nurse educator responds. *Nursing Outlook, 8*(10), 543–545.

Meleis, A. (1988). Doctoral education in nursing: Its present and future. *Journal of Professional Nursing, 4,* 436–446.

Moccia, P. (1986). DNS debate. *Nursing and Health Care,* 265.

Murphy, J. (1981). Doctoral education in, of, and for nursing: An historical analysis. *Nursing Outlook, 29,* 645–648.

Newman, M. A. (1975). The professional doctorate in nursing: A position paper. *Nursing Outlook, 23*(11), 704–706.

Pitel, M., & Vian, J. (1975). Analysis of nursing doctorates. *Nursing Research, 24,* 340–351.

Rogers, M. (1966). Doctoral education in nursing. *Nursing Forum, 5,* 75–82.

Schlotfeldt, R. (1978). The professional doctorate: Rationale and characteristics. *Nursing Outlook, 26*(5), 302–311.

Sherwin, L., Bevil, C., Adler, D., & Watson, P. (1993). Education for the future: A national survey of nursing deans about need and demand for nurse researchers. *Journal of Professional Nursing, 9*(4), 195–203.

Seitz, P. (1987). The pros and cons of doctoral education. *The Canadian Nurse* (May), 27.

Snyder-Halpern, R. (1986). Nursing doctorates: Is there a difference? *Nursing Outlook, 34,* 284–286.

Starck, P., Duffy, M., & Vogler, R. (1993). Developing a nursing doctorate for the 21st century. *Journal of Professional Nursing, 9*(4), 212–219.

Stevenson, J. S., & Woods, N. F. (1986). Nursing science and contemporary science: Emerging paradigms, in G.E. Sorenson (ed.), *Setting the agenda for the year 2000: Knowledge development in nursing.* Kansas City, MO: American Academy of Nursing.

Werley, H., & Leske, J. (1988). Pinning down the tracks to doctoral degrees. *Nursing and Health Care, 9,* 239–243.

Ziemer, M., Brown, J., Fitzpatrick, M. L., Manfredi, C., O'Leary, J., & Valiga, T. (1992). Doctoral programs in nursing: Philosophy, curricula, and program requirements. *Journal of Professional Nursing, 8*(1), 56–62.

CHAPTER THREE

On Curriculum

Doctoral education in nursing should be a tremendously broadening experience, as well as one that allows you to develop a focused area of expertise.

Student comment

INTRODUCTION

CURRICULAR ISSUES AT THE doctoral level, for students, center around research preparation, role preparation, interdisciplinary study and the development of writing and critical thinking skills. This chapter speaks to these issues both from the perspective of the student and in relationship to that which has been published in the literature. Interestingly, some of what is addressed in relationship to curriculum is tied directly to issues surrounding degree type. Although nursing continues to offer the PhD, DNS, and EdD, the curriculums have been found to be very similar.

Core curricular content identified as essential in doctoral programs includes "nursing theory, theory development, concept formulation and quantitative analysis" (Beare, Gray, Ptak, 1981, p. 314). Other relevant content includes "experimental design, research, ethics in health, legislation issues, trends and issues, nursing ethics, publishing, political issues and grantsmanship" (Beare et al., 1981, p. 314). "Computer instruction, health care delivery, role theory, accountability, change theory, resource planning, health, wellness, systems theory, stress theory, leadership theory, role socialization, and quality assurance" were identified as important concepts that should be included in a doctoral program (Beare et al., p. 313).

Currently, there are no specific mandated standards for doctoral education although the American Association of Colleges of Nursing (AACN, 1987, p. 72) has endorsed the curricular components that follow and considers these to be essential to any doctoral program:

a. History and philosophy and their relation to the development of nursing knowledge;

b. Existing substantive nursing knowledge;

c. Theory construction;

d. Social, ethical, and political issues of importance to the discipline.

e. Research designs, methods and techniques of analysis appropriate to the level of doctoral study;

f. Data management, tools, and technology; and

g. Student research opportunities.

RESEARCH FOCUS: THE QUANTITATIVE/ QUALITATIVE DEBATE

Research preparation at the doctoral level is viewed not only by those individuals responsible for the development and implementation of doctoral programs, but also by students, as the cornerstone to this level of education. The purpose of the doctoral degree is primarily to prepare research scholars and to certify that a student has demonstrated research competence in a particular discipline (Moore & Sacchetti, 1987). Development of a research background and the ability to conduct research is the central focus of all programs, whether one is talking about the PhD, DNS, or EdD in nursing.

Ziemer and colleagues (1992) reported on a study that examined the philosophy, curricula, and program requirements of doctoral programs in nursing. The authors noted that "empirical research has documented few distinguishing features among the various types of degree programs" (Ziemer et al., 1992, p. 57). Research and scholarship were identified as the expected outcome for graduates of all programs participating in this study. The authors further noted:

> Doctoral curricula in nursing also reflect an emphasis on quantitative research methodologies because only 16 of the doctoral programs explicitly included qualitative methodologies in their programs. Faculties who generate doctoral nursing curricula seem to have an affinity for emphasizing "hard science" (quantitative) methodologies.

This particular finding by Ziemer and colleagues (1992) is well noted by the participants in the study reported in this book and is supported by the narrative comments included at the end of the chapter. As one participant noted:

> Quantitative research is overemphasized. Mixed messages are given in that verbally qualitative studies are encouraged but students are expected to perform quantitatively in most courses.

According to the study conducted by Ziemer and colleagues (1992) only 16 out of 44 doctoral programs offered a qualitative research course.

Dennis (1991) offered a very clear description of what should be required in doctoral programs in order to ensure success in the clinical nurse researcher role. The central areas focused on were knowledge within the role of nursing, philosophy and ethics, research methodology, statistics, measurement, grantsmanship and dissemination of the research findings. Although Dennis (1991) addressed the specifics of preparing for a role as a clinical nurse researcher her comments really pertain to the research role for any nurse prepared at the doctoral level. If nursing is to gain credibility in academic settings her recommendations apply to the preparation of faculty nurse researchers as well. Dennis emphasized the need to familiarize oneself with a diversity of research designs and recommended that "doctoral programs that are strong across the qualitative-quantitative continuum will give the clinical nurse researcher the strong methodological background that is crucial for success in the role" (Dennis, 1991, p. 161).

Dennis (1991) further emphasized the need for students to be actively involved in research under the supervision of an experienced investigator. She advocated the need to work on more than just the dissertation and that to truly understand and develop in the researcher role one must be working at a minimum as a research assistant so that experience is obtained working on more than one research project.

A further consideration for nurse researchers is the development of the ability to complete statistical analysis of data and methods of measurement. Dennis (1991) noted that "a strong knowledge of statistics is a common weakness, both in nursing and in other fields" (Dennis, 1991, p. 162).

> Journals are replete with research reports where investigators analyzed complex, multivariate experimental designs with repeated applications of T-tests or lengthy iterations of other types of univariate analyses. As it develops its cadre of scientists, nursing does not need to prolong and perpetuate these inadequacies in the use of statistics (Dennis, 1991, p. 162).

Clinical nurse researchers as well as academic researchers need skills of data transfer and computerization. These include:

> The ability to develop code books and procedures for coding data, establish routines to enhance coding accuracy, set up computer files, write programs in the format of mainframe computer software applications such as SPSS, SAS, and BMDP, and/or use statistical software designed for microcomputers (Dennis, 1991, p. 162).

Meleis (1992) also discussed research preparation and strategies for the development of scholarship in doctoral students. She, like Dennis (1991) noted that the environment of doctoral study must stimulate scholarship and that the development of a scholar requires more than course work.

Students participating in the study included in this book noted in their narrative comments that they were prepared for the conduct of research. Most participants noted that they were prepared to conduct quantitative inquiries. The concerns and considerations voiced by participants in the study reported in this book are verified by Dennis (1991). Although students recognized that the purpose of doctoral education in nursing was to be prepared for the researcher role, the process is only a beginning. Many had hoped for more opportunity to be mentored and to work on an individual basis with faculty to improve their research skills.

Sherwin and colleagues (1993) discussed the importance of producing doctorally prepared nurse researchers capable of meeting the profession's unique research demands. In their national survey of nursing deans the research emphasis most highly valued was in the psychosocial domain. There was a belief that current and future funding potential was greatest for biophysical researchers.

Doctoral students participating in the study results included in this text believed that their programs had as their primary goal the preparation of scholars to conduct research. Doctoral education prepared them to raise appropriate questions, conduct research and to think critically although the true learning came after the degree in the actual conduct of research. Several participants noted that although their curriculums included research courses, they felt unable to conduct research without some input from a statistician. Students believe their research backgrounds at the doctoral level must be rigorous and that they need to be prepared to function in a competitive way with other academic and clinical researchers. The following student comments emphasize this point:

> Whether one chooses a quantitative or qualitative study, one should be exposed on a rigorous basis to both types of methodology and computer analysis of data.

> Doctoral education needs to be rigorous in preparing students for research, and expectations of the quality of dissertations needs to be high.

PREPARATION FOR WHAT? PRACTICE, EDUCATION, ADMINISTRATION AND/OR RESEARCH

Role preparation related to practice, education, and/or administration at the doctoral level is a secondary consideration to the goal of preparing nurse researchers. Anderson (1989) noted that what originally brought nurses to academic settings was the fact that they liked to teach. As the role of the nurse educator expanded in these settings, faculty were then required to earn doctorates and develop research agendas. Emphasis was placed on the need to develop master teachers and "to build research programs designed around clinical problems so our science will make a difference" (Anderson, 1989, p. 171).

Fitzpatrick (1991) also addressed role preparation at the doctoral level and much like Anderson (1989) advocated faculty preparation as both researcher and teacher. She emphasized, however, the need to develop researchers at the doctoral level as a first priority, allowing teaching, although critical, to come as a secondary role that can be developed in a faculty position. The role of teaching in many instances may fall to the employing institution in the opinion of Fitzpatrick (1991). The majority of doctoral programs in nursing have adopted curricular patterns that provide for substantial research preparation as a primary concern, few have addressed role preparation (Ziemer et al., 1992).

Fitzpatrick (1991) further emphasized the need to avoid reinforcing the following negative ideas:

1. that teaching in undergraduate education is less important and prestigious than graduate education;
2. that the ultimate goal of doctorally prepared faculty is graduate teaching;
3. that undergraduate teaching—especially clinical teaching—should be relegated to lesser prepared people or graduate assistants;
4. that teaching is secondary to research in the career of an academician;
5. that service to the university is routine, mundane, and not relevant to promotion or tenure decisions; and
6. that scholarly inquiry cannot be compatible with the role of undergraduate teaching in smaller, less research-oriented institutions (Fitzpatrick, 1991, p. 175).

In the study conducted by Ziemer and colleagues (1992) 22 out of 44 programs focused on role preparation for nurses.

> Role preparation was defined by the investigators as a nonclinical program with emphasis on preparation for a particular employment focus. Nine programs offered role preparation in educational administration, 10 in curriculum development, 18 in nursing administration, and 3 had a focus on preparation for a consulting role. Programs that focused on role preparation for doctoral education usually had two separate tracks for study. Sixteen of the doctoral programs offered both clinical and role preparation, and 14 schools did not specify either (Ziemer et al., 1992, p. 58).

Results of the quantitative data analysis reported in this book, as conducted by the authors, found that when doctoral students were asked if the doctorate prepared them for a specific role, i.e., researcher, practitioner, educator or administrator, PhD students had significantly different scores than EdD and DNS students. PhD students did not perceive the doctorate as a degree that prepared them for roles as educators, practitioners or administrators, but as researchers. In addition, PhD students did not view EdD and DNS programs as educational pathways that prepared students to engage in research. DNS students reported that research, specifically, quantitative research, was not a primary focus of their programs.

Narrative responses regarding role preparation addressed issues related to preparation as a researcher, educator, practitioner, and administrator. Students enrolled in doctoral programs, whether DNS, PhD, or EdD, believed that they were adequately prepared to conduct research in the majority of cases. Students enrolled in DNS and EdD programs perceived role preparation to be dual, as opposed to students enrolled in PhD programs who generally believe that they have a single focus . . . preparation as a nurse researcher. DNS students believe that their programs prepare them as researchers and expert practitioners while EdD students believe they are prepared as researchers and educators. Although some participants indicated that their career paths would lead to an administrative focus, this particular area of role preparation received the fewest comments.

There was some sense that more attention should be paid at the doctoral level to the preparation for faculty roles. Students noted that teaching excellence was not necessarily a concern of faculty at the doctoral level and that a weakness of PhD programs is that they fail to adequately prepare students to be educators. One student noted that "it would be helpful to be prepared as a teacher as well as researcher." Finally, students seemed to feel the pressures that come with life at the doctoral level. Sustaining a constant research focus with the ever present reminder that one must also maintain excellence in teaching, community service and publishing in order to retain faculty positions, may be overwhelming and/or impossible for some.

Selected student comments related to role preparation included:

Schools that have particular resources should develop concentrations in practice/research and education/research.

Advanced degrees prepare nurses for many other roles among which may be deanship, educator or practitioner.

The purpose of doctoral education is to prepare scholars—whatever their particular interests are for knowledge generation.

Part of what nursing education is about is promoting the profession through development of future researchers, leaders and educators.

Preparation for the roles of educator or administrator should be included in doctoral programs in nursing.

Not every nurse who pursues a doctoral degree plans to be a researcher.

The primary focus of doctoral education in nursing programs should be the preparation of nurse researchers and theorists-scholars.

Role preparation related to clinical practice issues is another area of concern as perceived by students participating in this study. Those doctoral students clearly grounded in practice believe that real advancement in nursing as a profession and discipline will not occur if we do not maintain our commitment to the practice arena. Pertinent narrative comments included:

> Emphasis to a much greater degree should be placed on advanced clinical knowledge development including the physical, biological, medical, psychological and sociological aspects of the profession.

> Educators need to be more fully engaged in clinical practice.

> Doctoral programs are not prepared to handle nurses who are in the clinical setting. They cannot believe a doctoral student could actually be functioning as a staff nurse.

> My clinical practice will be last and more importantly, I'm not being prepared to teach. I feel like I'm educating myself out of the role I love.

> Practice—that's where the theory-research-practice circle will be accomplished.

Narrative comments from students also indicated that there is some sense that doctoral preparation is really unrelated to preparation as an expert clinician or practitioner and that this type of preparation should remain at the Master's level. Narrative comments from students related to this line of thinking included:

> Clinical preparation should not be included in doctoral programs at all.

> The Master's degree is the clinical degree; advanced nursing is enhanced with a strong research and theory background gained at the doctoral level.

> Master's education is the proper place for the preparation of expert clinicians.

> Doctoral programs do not prepare excellent practitioners.

INTERDISCIPLINARY COURSE WORK

Courses from a variety of disciplines, as well as deliberative networking among faculty and students, are important aspects of doctoral education. In relationship to research, Dennis (1991) noted:

> The clinical nurse researcher who demonstrates expertise in statistical analysis and measurement, as well as skills in education and consultation, is bound to be recognized and sought by colleagues in other disciplines. This type of interdisciplinary interaction gives nurses important credibility as researchers and scientists, as well as professionals in the health care arena (Dennis, 1991, p. 163).

Narrative comments from students engaged in doctoral education indicated a strong sense that courses taken outside the major were necessary to broaden the educational experience and to provide exposure to experts in specific areas. This is particularly important when examining statistics requirements. Narrative comments from students indicated that these courses are primarily taken outside of the department and that they should remain so in order to maintain rigor. Students noted:

> Statistical methods taught outside the school of nursing have been much more rigorous and meaningful in my doctoral education.

> At least some classes taken out of the major discipline, be it nursing or whatever, are important to a more complete education.

> The elective courses I took in a number of other disciplines deepened and broadened my doctoral education.

> Courses in philosophy should be a part of all doctoral education in nursing.

> Statistics, as a support course, should be taught by statisticians, not by nursing faculty.

DEVELOPING WRITING SKILLS

Opportunities to publish and write grants are viewed by students as extremely important to the doctoral preparation. As one student noted:

> The opportunities for personal growth, e.g., through writing, publishing, and presenting have kept me motivated throughout the ordeal of studying quantitative research.

Many students find that opportunities for publishing and grant writing come after the doctorate and these opportunities are often left behind after graduation. Post doctoral work is viewed as important but not a realistic commitment for many given their family and work obligations.

CRITICAL THINKING SKILLS

All courses in a doctoral program should require and facilitate the student's ability to think clearly, logically, and critically. Consideration of all the possible approaches and issues to the study of nursing phenomena must be fostered in doctoral curriculums.

> Healthy classroom interchange and challenge among faculty and students promotes the ability to articulate and define ideas. Seemingly in a constant quest for perfection, the initial reaction to challenge may be to retreat from one's position, surmising that the other person is right, particularly when that person is senior and more experienced. But even imperfect positions and imperfect research proposals can be defended within the acknowledgment of limitations. Challenge stimulates growth and ideas within the scientific community, and it is important for doctoral students in nursing to learn to respond positively to it (Dennis, 1991, p. 164).

Narrative comments from students indicated that the development of their critical thinking abilities was an important component of doctoral education. This particular cognitive ability was developed as a result of classroom discussion with students and faculty and with opportunities to question the status quo, write, and perhaps publish. One participant commented:

> If nurses are to be critical thinkers, to synthesize knowledge and generate knowledge through research and publication, then didactic teaching should be limited, if not restricted, at the doctoral level. Rather, European style seminars, tutorials, case method and analysis should be utilized for adult learners.

SUMMARY

Doctoral education in nursing can be expected to grow and continue to emphasize research preparation as the primary focus. Similarities among the three types of doctoral programs suggests that there is agreement among nurse educators regarding the knowledge required at the doctoral level despite differences in labels.

Role preparation in terms of teaching, practice and administration continues to be a secondary concern. Although many programs, in particular DNS programs, emphasize role preparation, preparing scholars to conduct research is the primary agenda of most curriculums at the doctoral level.

NARRATIVE STUDENT COMMENTS RELATED TO RESEARCH PREPARATION

The didactic content related to research, particularly quantitative research was fairly strong and is improving.

Emphasis remains on quantitative research methods.

Heavily quantitative in its research focus.

A strong emphasis in research design and data evaluation—particularly quantitative analysis is provided.

There is preparation, acceptance and support for both qualitative and quantitative methodologies.

One continuing issue is the recognition of all approaches to research; qualitative and quantitative.

I conducted historical research which personally taught me a great deal.

I have learned to appreciate all approaches (quantitative and qualitative).

I'm a qualitative researcher at a research university—a quantitative research university. I have to work twice as hard to be viewed as credible.

Ten years ago I was not allowed to use qualitative research, which was the only appropriate method for my interest.

PhD nursing programs need to move toward inclusion of qualitative research emphasis.

At the master's and or doctoral level there is an inequity between quantitative and qualitative methods.

I think too little emphasis is placed on qualitative research techniques, especially qualitative analysis.

I have had to seek out a mentor to train me in qualitative techniques.

My hope is that qualitative research becomes as valued as quantitative.

Focus on both qualitative and quantitative methodologies in nursing research.

The lack of clinical emphasis seems to me to be a major omission of the PhD program.

I had no idea that research was the major focus of a nursing PhD—might not have started if I had known.

The doctoral program I attend emphasizes and prepares researchers in whichever method they choose. There is no qualitative/quantitative split.

The experience with research in my doctoral program was poor and not well guided. I had very little contact with faculty. Getting to see faculty required a major effort. I got more support from faculty outside the nursing department. Most of what I know about research and teaching, I learned on my own after I got my degree.

Research is important, but not at the expense of teaching.

The clinical focus must not be lost. Three years of academic without intermittent clinical work leaves a graduate far behind when returning to the "real" world. Exposure to other disciplines is important. I appreciated my EdD (which I chose over a PhD) because I did not focus narrowly, but took courses which enriched me.

I am not confident in doing research as a result of my doctoral education. I made every mistake possible—14 page questionnaire, 7 sections—it was the equivalent of 7 dissertations simultaneously. It was an overwhelming ordeal. I have not wanted to attempt anything since (ten years).

References

American Association of Colleges of Nursing (1987). Indicators of quality in doctoral programs in nursing. *Journal of Professional Nursing, 3,* 72–74.

Anderson, C. A. (1989). This isn't what I expected: The changing landscape of nursing education. *Journal of Professional Nursing, 5*(4), 171, 236.

Beare, P. G., Gray, C. J., & Ptak, H. F. (1981). Doctoral curricula in nursing. *Nursing Outlook, 29,* 311–316.

Dennis, K. E. (1991). Components of the doctoral curriculum that guide success in the clinical nurse researcher role. *Journal of Professional Nursing, 7*(3), 160–165.

Fitzpatrick, M. L. (1991). Doctoral preparation versus expectations. *Journal of Professional Nursing, 7*(3), 172–176.

Meleis, A. I. (1992). On the way to scholarship: From master's to doctorate. *Journal of Professional Nursing, 8*(6), 328–334.

Moore, T. C., & Sacchetti, R. D. (1987). *Graduate and professional programs: An overview 1987.* Princeton, NJ: Peterson's Guides.

Sherwin, L. N., Bevil, C. A., Adler, D., & Watson, P. G. (1993). Educating for the future: A national survey of nursing deans about need and demand for nurse researchers. *Journal of Professional Nursing, 9*(4), 195–203.

Ziemer, M. M., Brown, J., Fitzpatrick, M. L., Manfredi, C., O'Leary, J., & Valiga, T. M. (1992). Doctoral programs in nursing: Philosophy, curricula, and program requirements. *Journal of Professional Nursing, 8*(1), 56–62.

CHAPTER FOUR

On Mentoring

Be ever ready to praise, to encourage, to stimulate, but slow to censure, and still more slow to condemn.

Catherine McAuley

INTRODUCTION

EVERY NURSE SHOULD HAVE a mentor and every nurse should mentor. We have learned over the years that many successful people in various career paths have been influenced by a significant other. A protector, benefactor, coach or someone that served to build a dream in one's life. Someone who praised, encouraged and stimulated. Someone who critiqued but was slow to censor and in the words of Catherine McAuley, even slower to condemn. Artists have advised the apprentice on the techniques of watercolors. The ballerina has learned from the prima. The mason and carpenter pass down their trade and method. Successful athletes have mentors. Where would cyclist Greg LeMond be without his coach Eddie Borysewicz?

Nurses, every day in the clinical setting mentor other nurses on old and new techniques. Each day a bit of learning is passed down in our profession. In academia it is the same. The more experienced professor guides the novice on every level, baccalaureate, master's and doctoral preparation. It is a process of giving of self and selecting the protege with the best match. For the novice it is an intense desire to learn and take risks.

This chapter addresses the many attributes of the mentoring process. Personality characteristics, qualities and the significance of the mentoring experience both as mentor and mentee are addressed. For doctoral students mentoring is a significant aspect of their learning experience. Contemporary literature and the voices of doctoral students who participated in this study are addressed. The mentoring experience is an inspiring one and the void that is felt when this opportunity is absent in doctoral education is evident in student comments.

WHAT IS MENTORING?

The definition of mentoring has been noted in the nursing literature and discussed in many publications. Kelly (1984) differentiated between *mentors, sponsors* and *role models.*

> *Mentorship* itself is an intense relationship calling for a high degree of involvement between a novice in the field and the person knowledgeable and very powerful in the area. A mentor is a protector, supporter, teacher, and counselor, who eases the neophyte's entry and advancement into the work world, who initiates the protege into that world's unique values, customs, and cast of characters. *Sponsors* are strong patrons, but are less powerful than mentors in promoting and shaping proteges' careers. A *role model* or preceptor is not necessarily a mentor, but the mentor is almost always a role model and preceptor (p. 7).

> Fagan and Fagan (1983) view a mentor as an "experienced adult who befriends and guides a less experienced adult" (p. 77).

Hamilton (1981) noted:

> No two mentorships are ever the same but what occurs quite naturally is tutelage and guidance. Whether they are actual architects of dreams or helpers in the execution of the protege's dream, they somehow communicate the importance of dream making, career planning and strategy, and owning one's conception of career designing and putting it into perspective within their profession (p. 5).

Vance (1982) emphasized that mentoring is a "process by which an older, wiser, and more experienced person guides and nurtures a younger one—it is as old as the bonds between parent and child, master and disciple, teacher and student" (p. 7). In her research on the mentor relationship, Vance found that mentoring in nursing did occur and that 83 percent of influential nurses had someone they mentored and that most of the mentors were other nurses. A few examples of the benefits mentees received included career advice, guidance, scholarly stimulation, teaching, advising and emotional support.

A mentor is "someone who shares with the mentee the secrets of her or his success. This is often referred to as helping someone learn the ropes of the trade" (Cameron, 1982, p. 19). A mentoring relationship provides many of the same elements that are found in other guiding relationships such as advising, counseling and role modeling. The difference is that the mentor relationship goes beyond these other relationships (p. 20).

The mentoring relationship is not new to our profession. Nurses have mentored other nurses since the days of Nightingale. Communication skills, the leadership trade, nursing implementations and skills such as venipuncture have been passed down to the protege. Fagan and Fagan (1983) noted that mentoring is not a "lost art" in nursing and mentoring among nurses is better than other occupations such as law enforcement and teaching. Mentoring for "success," however, is a slow entity in the nursing profession (Davidhizar, 1988; Moore & Salimbene, 1981). Mentors for women in high profile careers are scarce (Sheehy, 1976; Vance, 1982). Mentors are vital and desperately needed in the profession to nurture students and future leaders.

Moore and Salimbene (1981) studied mentoring relationships and found that two major types of interactions occur—the superior/subordinate or older experienced one and younger inexperienced employee and, the faculty member and student relationship. In the first type, the protege is assumed at some point to take the mentor's place and is "groomed for the position" (p. 56). In the second type (faculty member and most often doctoral student), many subjects experienced cold and uncaring advisors who were "intellectually outstanding but not personable" (p. 57). There was consensus that "special qualities" were necessary to mentor and that "status" within the organization was a needed ingredient.

QUALITIES OF GOOD MENTORS

A good mentor must take a personal interest in the mentee, be able to share, coach and be, in essence, a good friend and role model. A one-to-one tutelage with similar ideals and common research interests is expected. A keen ability to socialize the new disciple is essential. The mentor should be a respectable researcher—intelligent, humane, and one that commands respect as a researcher and as a scholar. A doctorally prepared faculty member with research and clinical sensitivity would be a good example of a mentor (Kim & Felton, 1986). Cameron (1982) viewed the mentor as someone that is approachable and respected for professional achievements (p. 21). White (1988) studied academic nurse administrators and concluded that the most beneficial personality characteristics of significant mentors included competence, intelligence, maturity, and sincerity.

Lou Gerstner, chairman of the computer giant IBM has been a strong mentor to many management executives in the firm. IBM, having a disastrous 1994 in the personal computer business, has changed the management attitude under the mentorship of Gerstner.

> What I've found in IBM is that the very core strengths had always been there and were still there . . . the problem was more the attitudes, the kind of management structure and the management behavior that got built up in the face of success. I call it the curse of success (Newsweek, 1995, p. 120).

The good mentor is "approachable" by the mentee in Cameron's view (1982). It is someone the mentee respects or someone that you could go to with your concerns. The mentor is just there when you need her. For doctoral students the good mentor gives the notion of "come on in" rather than "do not disturb."

The good mentor cultivates, presents affiliations, pushes, tests, evaluates. They are available, organized and quite good at juggling multiple parts of life. For doctoral students good mentors first need to be approachable, and certainly available. The mentor is a conductor that orchestrates the many aspects of the doctoral process. Many doctoral students don't want much . . . trust, accomplishment of goals and tasks, and a road map that assists in completion of their work. Their narrative comments emphasize this point.

> I am getting a first class education. I can pick and choose my own program and minor courses so that they are tailor made for my career goals. The mentoring situation is excellent. The faculty are very available to meet. The course work is high quality.

> I've been adopted by my minor department in Sociology. My dissertation is guided by both departments. This has provided me with expert mentors from two areas. Our nursing program is new and the nursing faculty have not had a lot of experience guiding dissertations. My co-chair in Sociology is a pro with much experience at helping PhD candidates. These two factors have been the best experiences of my whole program.

> At my school there are large differences in the experiences of students depending on the contact with faculty members and mentors. I have a wonderful mentor (co-advisor) who is very interested in providing me with pertinent and helpful experiences as well as offering support and encouragement and being a great role model. I am actively working on a large NIH multi-site study, thus gaining hands on experience in conducting research which is helping me in my own work. This has not been the case for all students and I feel fortunate to have this experience.

> My mentor has coached me through every step of the research process—from grant application to publication of results.

> It is essential that there be a strong professional relationship between doctoral faculty and graduate students with personal support through the rugged periods . . . essential also is to have doctoral candidates

actively participating in research and publication with doctoral faculty members before graduation.

Genuine mentors expect to be involved with students.

QUALITIES OF GOOD MENTEES

The mentee must also possess certain qualities. The mentee must have a strong desire to learn, work hard and most importantly have a "good attitude." The mentee must trust the mentor and go to the mentor for direction (Cameron, 1982). Mentees must be willing— willing to socialize into the network or affiliation; willing to take the ups and downs that are part of success or leadership. The mentee must be bright, not brilliant, but be willing to go the extra yard to learn and be prepared at a moment's notice to change and invite change.

Self assurance is a vital quality of a good mentee. Many students, for example, are afraid to ask questions or challenge the experienced leader for the sake of learning. They lack personal confidence and self-esteem. They want to model the mentor but lack the finesse and experience to do so.

For female mentees, obstacles that affect women must additionally be considered. These include being unmarried and the pressure to marry, postponement or elimination of childbearing, and being perceived in the female stereotype and labeled "too emotional" (Sheehy, 1976). There is also the public perception that when females are mentored by males there is a sexual component to the relationship.

The following anecdotes by Booth (1994) illustrate an example of a good mentoring and good mentee episode:

> A close friend of mine who often complains about his teaching failures decided one year to "put his all" into a year-long freshman class, with the specific assignment to himself to ensure that as many students as humanly possible should survive in good shape into the sophomore year. "What better measure of success," he was fond of

asking his colleagues, "than whether students at the end of the year are still there, both wanting to continue and able to continue, because they now have the necessary equipment (including a certain amount of misguided pride) for becoming sophomores?" He met with his class during the regularly scheduled period each week but also added a writing tutorial each week. "His agenda was to prove to the administration that if every freshman had at least one such class, experiencing ardent attention not just to reading and writing but to personal anxieties and deficiencies, the drop-out rate could be drastically reduced" (p. 34).

So then a good mentor is creative, dedicated and equips the student with the skills needed to succeed. The leader is also perceptive to the needs of the neophyte that impact upon academe. Attention to both emotional and psychological needs in the above scenario were demonstrated, and attention to the skills as well as attitudes were provided in a caring framework. It is therefore, the bigger picture which must be addressed. The mentor must not only provide mentees with the tools of the trade, the mentor must act on hunches and be able to assess humanness. The mentor must be in tune behaviorally to problems that occur and affect the mentoring episode. Good mentees will then follow the lead and persevere. This "followship" only happens because the mentor cultivated a flicker into a flame and inspired the mentee's hard work.

WHAT ARE BAD MENTORS? TOO LITTLE OR TOO MUCH

First of all, mentors don't plan to ever be bad mentors. They may be very caring people who are "overindulged" in the work setting as administrators, academics or clinicians. Often beyond the mentors' control are many masters and commitments. However, mentors can offer too little to their mentees.

The mentee on the other hand is literally blind to the warning signs of overworked mentors. It is key to be aware of these signs as a mentee so a better mentor match occurs (if it is within your control). Mentees are in the "me-me" stage when looking for a mentor. They are very needy and vulnerable at this point and they just want a mentor, anyone. They cannot differentiate between mentors that are too busy or not too busy. Where does that leave the nurse mentee? Be aware of the warning signs of mentors that have a full plate:

   a. They never answer your phone calls.
   b. They are frequently interrupted when you are in conference with them.
   c. They call you "Mary" when your name is "Jane."
   d. They lack a sense of humor.
   e. They are uninspiring.
   f. They frequently talk about their own needs.
   g. They are absorbed in their own research.
   h. They don't have a life.
   i. They philosophically focus on a cup that is half empty rather than half full.

Too little "contribution" translates to not being available when the student is in need. Rather than protecting, the mentor allows the protege to flounder in a sea of insecurity. There is no coaching, orchestrating, or sponsoring. Not being honest when workload, family, and research are the priority rather than the needs of the mentee, develops into a dysfunctional relationship. In nursing, we are often guilty of "too little." Nurse faculty have many hidden agendas, some of which are so inherent in the work they do that they probably do not realize the juggling that occurs. . . . committees, professional organization commitments, overload scheduling, too many advisees . . . and the list goes on. Doctoral students noted:

> My life changed dramatically as I found myself a single mother with five young children, which necessitated my return to graduate school for my master's degree. Achieving my PhD represents a significant personal and professional goal for me. My children have cheered me

on. Unfortunately, my most significant support and mentoring has not come from the faculty in the institution where I am completing my doctorate, but rather from co-workers where I teach, and from my peers in the doctoral programs.

Part of what nursing education is about is promoting the profession through development of future researchers, leaders and educators. I have found that while this tenet is spoken about it is not a focus of the actions. The system seems to have lost its focus. The focus is now individual pursuits whether they be tenure, research, money or notoriety. I have been somewhat discouraged by that and am uncertain whether I will continue in nursing higher education or pursue a clearly new vision of how education can benefit the discipline.

My professional and personal growth during my doctoral education, specifically with regard to self confidence, has been mostly a result of my own initiative and hard work rather than due to either faculty or curricular support. In fact, I have not found faculty at my institution to be particularly concerned with students' sense of self confidence, self esteem, or self respect.

I believe that a faculty mentor should be available to and accessible to all students. In my program, mentoring must be initiated by the student (which it should be); but should be more vigorously encouraged.

Personally, my support has come from my husband and other doctoral students. Faculty have given some support but they are so busy it is often hard to burden them with my need to "talk things out."

Very crucial to have mentorship; to establish a supportive relationship with a skilled researcher within one's area of interest. Haven't found that yet.

I wish there were more opportunities for a collegial relationship with faculty. Faculty continue to maintain their distance from relationships other than student-teacher. I see this as unfortunate for both.

I feel a tension and power struggle among the faculty and sometimes students are caught in the middle. My biggest disappointment is in faculty mentorship. I do not think I'm being provided the kind of mentoring that I anticipated doctoral education would have. Maybe my expectations were too high.

There is a lack of faculty mentorship of doctoral nursing students in general. In addition, the process of doctoral education, its goal of "reshaping" the individual, is destructive to self esteem.

Everything was smooth through candidacy then, it's been like being "thrown to the wolves."

I feel that faculty mentorship is an essential part of doctoral study. I was disappointed to find that this is not a value that is fostered in all doctoral programs. I was hoping to develop a mentoring relationship with my chairperson but that has not happened.

Faculty actively engaged in research and doctoral education are busy people. I found it difficult to connect with them at first. They were too busy. During my second semester, I was able to connect with faculty. I had to change my research focus, take an RA position, and explore faculty interests. I believe, prior to admission to the doctoral program that I needed a specified area of interest and at least a short track record in that arena. *Not true.* Rather, I needed to come to school, be open to faculty areas of interest and then seek a common ground.

During my doctoral studies, the support I have received has been 90–95 percent from other students in the program. Advisors don't have the time and professors don't take the time to get to know their students. Of course, there are exceptions, but the majority want to spend minimal time with students.

Faculty are completely out of touch with the reality of clinical nursing. This certainly does not enhance the relationship between theory, research and clinical practice. My own research interests and appreciation for a graduate education are intimately related to my clinical practice. Most faculty at our institution are too busy with their own research to teach. Personal and emotional support is nonexistent.

The other side of the coin is a phenomena called "overkill." The mentor actually gives too much. Similar to a flower drenched in water, the student is flooded with advice, not allowed to grow and essentially drowns, or worse—loses interest. Booth (1994) wrote:

Too much evidence of caring, too much individual attention is too much. If we swing from the chandeliers and tell joke after joke and hold many coffee hours or home visits, obviously more students will think we're great; they may even decide to become teachers too. But too much is too much, on both sides of a delicate balance; they will have been harmed if we've charmed them into a love of empty trickery (p. 34).

Overkill is not the idea of healthy mentoring. It is a balance that provides the student with enough trust and concern yet doesn't smother. The mentor sees the need for contributing but strikes a balance that allows growth and independence. Too much "contribution" can stifle the mentee if not scare one away.

White (1988) surveyed nurse administrators on the role of mentoring in career development and success. Many of the authors' findings fall into the "too much" category and nurses can really learn from this. Negative behaviors of mentors included provoking anxiety, being overly demanding of loyalty, manipulativeness and being overly possessive. Other negative behaviors included overdependence, treatment of the mentee as a token, limitation of career progress and transgression of sexual boundaries. Doctoral students noted:

> Faculty push the idea of socialization into the doctoral student role and ultimately the professional role of a doctorally prepared nurse. The reality today, with decreased funding, and increased need to be employed, family commitments, and commuting needs, sharply curtails full participation. It is inappropriate to be chastised for these realities.

> I believe that doctoral programs need to focus their specialties into two to three specific issues and recruit students who match these specific issues (or focuses). My program broadly accepted any student regardless of the student's interest and then could not "mentor" the student nor support the student in the dissertation process. A mentor/advisor needs to be established during the first year.

Balance is what the doctoral student should seek. Be aware of the warning signs of those who are not able to enable you. Look for someone who is honest about scholarly activities and time frames; a person who values your goals and assists you in attaining them.

BENEFITS IN THE MENTORING RELATIONSHIP

If the student or mentee can develop a successful relationship with a mentor, the benefits are plentiful. Sheehy (1976) linked mentors in the successful woman's life. She cited many pairs—and the impact of the mentors (mostly male) on the mentees (mostly female). Freud and Jung, Henry Higgins and Liza, Franz Boas and Margaret Mead, Jean-Paul Sartre and Simone de Beauvoir, Robert Browning and Elizabeth Barrett. She noted:

> There is no doubt that both mentor and apprentice reap enormous rewards from the association. It was Colette's first husband who literally sat her down in a room and told her to write. He had the contact; she was to be his instrument. For all his imperiousness, she did learn to write like a demon and eventually to do it on her own terms (p. 34).

Vance (1982) cited many rewards of the mentor relationship; preparation for leadership, career advancement and personal growth. She further noted that these relationships are especially important when career or life changes occur. A good mentor is there to assist in thinking through decisions and providing support and guidance. In academic settings mentorship is quite common. White (1988) concluded in a study of 300 academic nurse-administrators that all but 29 reported a mentoring connection of some sort. Mentoring, she emphasized was a "developmental" process that assisted one's career path. Initiating mentoring relations was either mutual or a role taken on by the mentor. It was also noted that personalities did not need to be similar for a successful relationship. Rawl and Peterson (1992) predicted level of career development of nursing education administrators. Mentored subjects published and received grant funding significantly more than nonmentored subjects. In addition, mentored subjects held doctorates more often than the nonmentored subjects.

The true mentoring benefits can be evaluated by the mentee achieving success, the mentor feeling accomplished, and both attaining a mutual benefit in goal attainment. In the voice of the student:

One of the outstanding aspects of my program is the support and facilitation that faculty give doctoral students. The message is: "grow, stretch, you can do it."

I feel that student-faculty mentorships are critical in doctoral education. Having been in both the situation of having and of not having a mentor, I can speak to the many advantages of having one. These include: networking with the mentor's colleagues, being a part of a research team, and being personally encouraged professionally and personally.

I did not limit myself to nursing courses in doctoral education—so many of my answers are based on the fact that I also received a certificate of women's studies during my doctoral course work. The courses I took and faculty I interacted with had a strong impact on my educational experience and contributed to many of the areas you asked about—such as my ability to be a critical thinker, the increase in my self confidence and the importance of networking with other students and faculty. I strongly encourage doctoral students to gain a more interdisciplinary education.

I am extremely impressed with my doctoral education. One experience that has greatly enhanced my education is having a mentor and going through the process of applying for a National Research Service Award. My mentor has coached me through every step of the research process, from a grant application to publication of results.

I believe one of the most important aspects of doctoral education is having a strong relationship with a mentor who can help you relate the education to real life. My original goal was to only complete my master's degree, but a professor with whom I developed a mentoring relationship helped me decide to continue with doctoral education. I think this contact truly decides the quality of a person's doctoral education.

BARRIERS IN THE MENTORING RELATIONSHIP

A closet of devils impede mentoring in nursing according to Hamilton (1981). Nurses and women have had difficulty initiating and

participating in mentoring because of their socialization as females—they were socialized *not* toward success as much as toward
belonging. Other factors impairing mentoring include: a lack of emphasis for women on team involvement and competition, it "not
being feminine" to succeed, a lack of full commitment to a career,
burn out, and reluctance. The author noted that many women have
struggled so much to be successful in their careers that they are
quite reluctant to guide a protege. Time is also another barrier.
Many women are so involved in committee activity, research and
"having a life" that little time exists to mentor. Doctoral students
have also felt the effects of the barriers in mentoring relationships
which may leave students quite frustrated, as can be seen in the
following narrative responses:

> Doctoral education has not met my expectations, especially this pro-
> gram. I expected a collegial environment between and among fac-
> ulty and students. Thus far, I have witnessed faculty that have ranged
> from incompetent to raving zealots. If I had to do it all over again, I
> would pursue a degree not in nursing. Several of my colleagues went
> this route and were more satisfied. Why is it that nursing education
> has to be so rigid and controlling?

> Colleges place faculty in the tenuous position of having to produce,
> leaving little time to spend mentoring students.

> Students should be able to change their sponsor when there is a
> conflict.

> Too often I know the horror stories about crazy faculty who are
> working out their own ego needs on doctoral students.

> I was my sponsor's first doctoral student. She made lots of mistakes
> and I suffered. She also had too many students, as well as her own
> teaching and research.

> When nursing faculty were not available as advisors, mentors were
> available in administration and research in other departments and
> other schools of nursing.

> Mentorship is simply a buzz word. It is not related to reality and
> hence not practiced.

> We should demonstrate the caring curriculum.

Gender was cited by Moore and Salimbene (1981) as a variable in mentoring. Their research indicated that males only had male mentors, and that male mentors had wider administrative exposure. Females had both male and female mentors. Female mentors were in traditional female roles such as a dean of a nursing school, dean of students or dean of women. In addition "cross-gender relationships" can be problematic. Social implications and how male/female relationships are perceived are barriers. Some mentor pairs are considered to be "having an affair" and some relationships are said to exceed professional parameters (p. 62).

DOCTORAL EDUCATION AND MENTORING: AN ESSENTIAL RELATIONSHIP

Although nursing has several hurdles to clear in its mentoring commitments, the need for mentoring is essential. Doctoral students benefit from a personal relationship that is focused on the mentee, yet, embraces the expertise and experiences of the knowledgeable teacher. Mutual respect, energy and quality performance are expectations on both sides of the mentee/mentor equation. Six specific ingredients of the mentoring relationship in doctoral education have been detailed by Davidhizar (1988): forward-mindedness (an orientation to the future), common interest (shared direction of what is essential), advice and strategies (toward goal attainment), self exposure (self-disclosure, trust, willingness), affirmation (enhance self-esteem), and how to mentor (the mentee shall mentor).

In terms of forward-mindedness, the ultimate goal is preparation for leadership—to learn the art of the leadership role in nursing. Both mentor and mentee must be enthusiastic about the present but look into the future.

The mentor and mentee should also have a common interest or a "shared sense of direction about what is important," that is, a similar direction in research, writing or public speaking. This translates into a most accomplished mentor. The mentee, however, has creativity and enthusiasm to share which provide "fresh vigor and stimulation" in the relationship. Both contribute and mutual change occurs.

Advice and strategy relates to the mentor showing the less experienced one the ropes. Because the mentor may have made mistakes in the past, advice and strategy toward goal attainment can occur. The big difference between the mentor and mentee is the past. "The mentor can provide critiques of both past and present actions of the mentee. In so doing, the mentor develops critical thinking and provides ideas which guide and shape the mentee's future actions" (p. 778).

On a more personal note Davidhizar (1988) refers to the concept, "self exposure." This characteristic has a few prerequisites: trust, self-disclosure, sensitivity, and willingness. It also requires that the mentor acknowledge the mentee's growth and provide earnest respect for the mentee's past accomplishments.

Affirmation is vital. The student is in an inferior role and affirmation by the mentor can enhance positive self-esteem. "For some mentors, facilitating someone else's growth results in more satisfaction than a more tangible success" (p. 780).

Finally, the characteristic of "mentees will be mentors" (Davidhizar, 1988, p. 782) was addressed. If one has had a good mentoring relationship it is likely that a positive relationship will recur when the mentee takes on the leadership role. The mentee may then be willing to take the chance and offer guidance to a less experienced nurse using the techniques and advice from their mentor.

The Voice of the Doctoral Student on Mentoring

Coming from another country (other than the United States) I am especially satisfied with the way the faculty accommodates assignments and works to suit the situation I came from and will return to. This does not mean they are lowering the requirements, rather the contrary, since I do have extensive education and experience in scholarly work in my home country. I enjoy the opportunity to stretch and strengthen my abilities in a highly scholarly environment.

Generally this faculty is open to a free debate with the students encouraging the individual's perspective.

Perhaps the strongest component of my doctoral education has been the combined effort of doctoral faculty to assist me in developing my ability to make logical connections when developing arguments and to use research to substantiate my ideas.

I feel one of the biggest issues in developing faculty at the doctoral level is strong mentoring. Faculty need to be guided in their professional development by ones who have gone before. This has been one of the strongest supports in my doctoral program and one that has helped me develop my future role as a doctorally prepared nurse.

I had an excellent experience personally but I don't know if it was due to an extensive clinical and teaching background, my own rather strong personality, the excellent faculty and advisors encountered or as I suspect a combination of all of these.

The peer/mentor relationship is critical to doctoral studies.

I attribute my professional success to the sound foundation offered me by extraordinary faculty.

In my program, each faculty member was a formidable nurse researcher who published in his/her own area.

Commitment of faculty to fostering of independence and risk taking.

Faculty believed in their students and in a sense became professional colleagues.

I believe that before embarking into doctoral education in nursing, one needs to design long-term goals and then choose a doctoral program that will assist with meeting those goals. For example, if I decide that my ultimate goal is to become a clinical nurse researcher, I should choose a doctoral program that will prepare me for this goal, not one that will prepare me to be an educator. Additionally, an important part of any doctoral program is faculty mentorship. If faculty are not available in the clinical or research area of interest to you, doctoral education becomes much more difficult. These mentoring relationships should be investigated prior to applying to a doctoral program.

I feel my program is one of the best in the country. The faculty as well as the Dean, are outstanding. Specifically, I've found the faculty supportive, kind, directive yet flexible. They have many part-time students (by the way, part-time programs need to be available) so we have many things going on in our individual lives (work, family, and school). I find the faculty to be incredibly understanding of this, yet maintain very high standards. The faculty are knowledgeable and have a broad understanding of the philosophy of science from different perspectives. I have found in talking to other doctoral students in other programs in the area, that we are receiving an exceptional education in terms of having a fair amount of exposure to some of the "newer" areas in science. Though it may sound funny, I have simply felt privileged to have this experience. It is energizing, challenging, and rewarding.

WEANING

What if a good relationship has occurred and continues to occur with a doctoral faculty member and a student? When is the time ripe for weaning from the relationship? Is it possible to separate?

It seems much like a parent who sets a child free—when they are mature and ready. So too must the mentor set the mentee free. This does not necessarily mean that the mentee must never be in touch with the mentor past graduation or job completion. It means that a strong bond or connection continues, but in a different framework. Good mentors keep in touch yet attend to their own aspirations. They are there, in the words of Vance (1982), many times in the transitional periods; such as a job change or career move. In these changing periods in one's life, a good mentor will be available to give advice, be frank and tell you that you are either making the biggest mistake of your life or missing the chance of a lifetime. Weaning must occur—if it does not then the relationship is stifled and not beneficial to either party. The mentee is stunted and the mentor controls. A doctorally prepared faculty member offered this example:

My mentor or doctoral faculty advisor was always there—maybe too much—helping me set deadlines, I feel, quite rigid deadlines, demanding better work, more narrative. She clearly had very high expectations. But after the dust settled and the dissertation was near, she let me go—defended my work to a committee of distinguished professors. I know she rather enjoyed my growth as a scholar during my dissertation defense . . . I still hear from her and I still call her—she is there when I need a critique of my writing or to offer advice and strategize—to make me see the forest through the trees. She causes me to introspect and evaluate my work until this day. She even sent me a copy of her new management text. That really impressed me—I feel fully weaned now—I am no longer a protege but a colleague.

I am glad to be given the opportunity to express in writing the issues that I see as important to doctoral education in nursing. I am somewhat unique in that I began the doctoral program at the age of 28, currently I am 31 years old, so the issues that are important to me may not be those of the majority of nursing doctoral students. I have completed my course work and comprehensive exams and am at the stage of writing the proposal for my dissertation. The role of faculty in the process of doctoral education is crucial to the output of the school. We have very strong faculty in our program, the majority of whom have ongoing funded research projects. I believe mentorship is crucial for those of us who are beginning researchers and a research assistantship is an excellent way to gain experience and a few extra dollars . . . I have found that the role of faculty gets somewhat nebulous once the course work is over. I have had little contact with the members of my dissertation committee since completion of my comprehensive exams. Once a student has completed course work, it is difficult to keep the ties with committee members.

SUMMARY

The main advantage that women, nurses, and doctoral students have is that sisterhood and guidance come quite naturally to many of us. It is what we do best and why so many of us became nurses in the first place. We have an ability to care and help those in need of our direction and concern. We need to appreciate the benefits of one-to-one mentoring and be aware of the barriers that impact our role. We also need to have a watchful eye on other professions, the successful ones that mentor the student into leader. If we succeed in mentoring, our mentoring will enable nursing leaders. "If mentoring is to find a home in nursing, we must understand our image of leadership and determine how its characteristics and traits can be cultivated through mentorship" (Hamilton, 1981, p. 10).

References

Booth, W. C. (1994). Beyond knowledge and inquiry to love, or: Who mentors the mentors? *ACADEME, 29–36.*

Cameron, R. K. (1982). Wanted: Mentor relationships within nursing administration. *Nursing Leadership, 5*(1), 18–22.

Davidhizar, R. E. (1988). Mentoring in doctoral education. *Journal of Advanced Nursing 13,* 775–781.

Fagan, M. M., & Fagan, P. D. (1983). Mentoring among nurses. *Nursing & Health Care,* 77–82.

Hamilton, M. S. (1981). Mentorhood: A key to nursing leadership. *Nursing Leadership, 4*(1), 4–13.

Kelly, L. (1984). From the president. *Sigma Theta Tau Reflections, 10*(7).

Kim, M. J., & Felton, G. (1986). Research mentoring. *Journal of Professional Nursing,* p. 142.

Moore, K. M., & Salimbene, A. M. (1981). The dynamics of the mentor-protege relationship in developing women as academic leaders. *Journal of Educational Equity and Leadership, 2,* 51–64.

Rawl, S. M., & Peterson, L. M. (1992). Nursing education administrators: Level of career development and mentoring. *Journal of Professional Nursing, 8*(3), 161–169.

Sheehy, G. (1976). The mentor connection. The secret link in the successful woman's life. *New York, 8,* 33–39.

Vance, C. N. (1982). The mentor connection. *The Journal of Nursing Administration, 12*(4), 7–13.

White, J. (1988). The perceived role of mentoring in the career development and success of academic nurse-administrators. *Journal of Professional Nursing, 4*(3), 178.

CHAPTER FIVE

On Networking

INTRODUCTION

MARY HIGGINS CLARK, the suspense novelist, once said, "If I were the mythical godmother, I would wish for you the joy of faith, wish and pray that you have special people in your lives, wish for you the ability to change what needs to be changed in the world, and wish for you a great sense of humor." In the nurse network, special people constantly enter our lives—the mythical godmothers are our mentors, and the special people are other students, family members and friends. These great relationships evolve for the doctoral student, and though many occur by chance, they may develop into lasting friendships and sources of support. The support is multi-faceted and often includes faculty, peers and programmatic support.

Students are basically happy with networking connections. Many have indicated that the relationships began as first-year students and were a "key" to successful completion of course work and dissertations. Others, however, wrote about stories of frustrations and a great deal of negativity.

The purpose of this chapter is to report how students perceive networking systems on the doctoral level. Verbatim anecdotes are presented from the view of the student. Many doctoral students throughout the country reported that networking is vital as one develops as a student, and later in professional nursing practice. Others feel that doctoral programs need to reevaluate and strengthen the support offered and continue to develop this essential part of doctoral education for nurses.

THE CONCEPT OF NETWORKING

Networking probably means many things to many people, but in the words of Robinson (1995):

> The basic purpose of networking is to improve one's personal and professional effectiveness. When applied to nursing, networking (or the utilization of contacts for information and advice) is an essential part of the process of developing and expanding a tested base of knowledge, which then constitutes and governs professional nursing practice (p. 262).

Networking does not just happen. It develops in phases as the student becomes socialized as a doctoral student and clearly, after graduation. For the student who is enrolled part time, it is vital to connect with colleagues and faculty. Every aspect of the networking process serves some purpose—where to park the car safely, sharing the notes on last week's empirical methods class, learning the meaning of extant theory in practice, or evaluating one's own place in the total equation.

The process has four dimensions as we see it: private (parallel play), participative (the comfort zone), personal (a friend), and at last, professional (a friend for life).

PARALLEL PLAY

Doctoral students network indirectly as early neophytes. It is a behind the scenes "getting to know you" pattern that originates in the classroom setting. Come to class—a brief hello, good bye, and see you next week. It can be envisioned as a type of parallel play where students are new and don't intensely interact but rather observe, listen, and of course, learn. Students at this level may find themselves outsiders. They may not know any other students or faculty, and may be unfamiliar with the city in which the program exists. They may have just survived a workday, a long commute, or a hassle finding a parking place. Although they may be hungry and possibly unpleasant, they continue to return because they are driven toward completing the goal of the doctorate. Each week they return to a pattern—same seat, observe, listen, learn. They often refrain from speaking and interacting because they are new and unknown. Faculty must realize that although many of these students are quite worldly and may be leaders within their organizations, the doctoral setting is intimidating and may thwart active participation for a considerable amount of time. This type of parallel observation lasts until doctoral students find a comfort zone.

> I have only started my doctoral program . . . I do, however, see the importance of peer support. I was immediately aware of how we support each other.

> Pursuing the doctorate has been truly a growth experience. I have become more adept at thinking critically and presenting ideas logically. In my first course, taught by a non-nurse philosopher, it was stated that we would all become premier researchers by the time we finished the program after five semesters of course work. This is becoming a reality. The curriculum is clearly focused and the faculty are very demanding. The program is always challenging yet supportive throughout. The collegial spirit among faculty and students is wonderfully stimulating. This is one of the best experiences of my life.

> My doctoral education is as much personal development as professional development. I learn almost as much from my student colleagues as I do from my instructors.

> At our school, networking and student support is really up to the student. That is probably fine at our level, but some assistance in initially organizing a networking set up would be helpful as most people don't know the system.

THE COMFORT ZONE

This phenomena in doctoral education occurs during the first year of collegial exchange. Students are now participative, have established a few student and faculty connections and become more involved in the group. They are also expected to be involved in group projects and presentations in the curricula. Relationships are being established and collegial trial and error occurs. Educators network with other educators for example, or clinicians with clinicians. What happens at this point is the beginning of relationships that may in fact last forever. Friendships are chosen and impact upon the student's life and career goals. Similar ideas become passions and may lead to shared research. Critique is respected and requested. It is a maturing that grows out of familiarity and supports growth.

> In my case, the need to feel that I legitimately belonged in such a well-respected program was the most outstanding issue to me. It took the whole first year of passing the preliminary exams before I obtained this sense of "OKness."

> Faculty were helpful and receptive to our ideas. They were skillful in guiding our thinking without loss of self-respect. While in classes, classmates were supportive of each other. Due to work and family commitments, we weren't able to get together often socially—if at all.

> Being doctorally prepared has reinforced why I love nursing and I want to share my love of the profession, not only with other nurses, but with the whole world. I don't think being doctorally prepared is an end to the means; to me it is only the beginning of learning more about nursing and all of its arms; practice, education, research, and administration.

> Pursuance of a PhD was based on my personal goals of improving my research preparation and establishing a professional network to facilitate research activities.

> Achieving my PhD represents a significant personal and professional goal for me. I have gained much from the experience and am now gathering data for my dissertation, so it seems achievable. My children have cheered me on. Unfortunately my most significant support and mentoring has not come from the faculty in the institution where I am completing my doctorate, but rather from co-workers where I teach and my peers in the doctoral program.

> I have found it vital to share and discuss anything and everything with other students. They are from all kinds of areas and backgrounds and often can see things in a way I can't.

The positive experiences in the PhD program have been:
a. close relationship with two faculty mentors.
b. strong emphasis on nursing science, including research.
c. collegiality with other doctoral students.

The faculty support and expertise is outstanding at my university. The stats and research courses are rigorous and they really prepare you to do research. The nursing administrative faculty and courses are superb. My classmates are now some of my best friends. There was great support for one another.

The most encouraging aspect has been the formation of friends within the doctoral program. At least fellow students (most) are supportive of their peers. I think if doctoral programs could empower their students, graduates would have a greater interest in pursuing additional post-doctoral study and research.

PERSONAL

Networking may become quite personal and enable relationships to solidify. Students learn more and more about each other, their lived experiences, families, fears, and become equipped with survival tools shared by others privy to the network. They may share family events along the way. They always share ideas about their profession in some way . . . over lunch . . . a bat mitzvah . . . a golf match. What occurs is a personal type of networking that lasts forever. This "personality" takes time to nurture and may not occur until the doctoral program is complete, but it does occur, and those who have experienced it know it and appreciate it.

Students' peer support is essential to survival at my school. We have a doctoral work area with adjacent computer lab and mainframe printer. This area facilitates the student support and provides us with our disks and files and a place from which to work.

Peer collegiality is the singular essential component that maintains the student's sense of worth throughout the program. It is likely that these will remain lifetime bonds. However, it is unfortunate that the rigor of doctoral studies must be made even more difficult by the self-doubt that attends students and is only slightly mediated by successful completion of candidacy. In many ways, it is a solitary endeavor, even while surrounded by family and friends.

Doctoral education has long been a goal for me. I love the intellectual exercise, aggressive networking and opportunity to challenge myself. For my purposes, doctoral education will position me to do research that is clinically based—to become a clinical nurse scientist. I want to know I've accomplished tasks that will enhance nursing practice.

PROFESSIONAL

The networking continues for the doctoral graduate. Professional networking is sophisticated and may take the shape of speaking engagements, post doctoral study, or shared writing projects. For example, the book that you both felt should be written, or the research project you envisioned can now occur. Many nurses at this point have raised their children, or just have more time available, and want to practice scholarship with the colleagues they have grown and matured with professionally. It is the last dimension of networking. It can be equated with a "tune in" type of atmosphere where true leadership and scholarship can be attained.

EXPRESSIONS OF NEGATIVITY

Despite the growth that many doctoral students report because of networking and peer support, many students were not positive about their experiences. Comments about competitive peers, unavailable faculty, and misleading deans seemed to have hampered networking attempts by students. This less than positive view, is essential to report. Doctoral programs are continuing to develop and strengthen nationwide and input from the voice of the student is important. Students enrolled in these programs have fresh and current views offering firsthand details as they lived the experience.

Those who have completed a doctorate know quite well that it is a most challenging time in one's life. We depend on support and some sort of pat on the back. Nurse networks and collegial sharing make it happen (completion of the doctorate).

We also know of those who have never finished—the "ABD" or all but dissertation group. Many know of someone who has not completed the doctorate in nursing. Granted, personal experiences, illness or life change are reasons why dissertations may not be completed. The profession needs to review support systems for doctoral nursing students, particularly those writing dissertations or nearing this point.

It is worth contemplating. Why does this happen? Why does it happen with relative frequency? The following comments suggest rationale for this "fall out" in the nursing community.

A real issue is the need for more opportunity to interact on an informal basis with both other doctoral students and faculty about research interests. Once one finishes with course work in particular, there is a drop in available social support and ability to describe research ideas with others (in the formative or conceptual phase). I have started my own informal network with students to discuss issues—it would be extremely helpful however, to have some type of seminar (non-graded perhaps) to discuss each other's research. It would certainly facilitate getting through the dissertation phase more readily and with less of a feeling of isolation.

My school is very good with respect to the formal aspects of doctoral education. They do not shine in terms of the informal, networking, mentoring aspects. I don't think this will change until faculty perceive they could get something from the students. At present, rubbing shoulders with students is something you do to "socialize" the students. It is not viewed as something that could help the faculty. When the faculty view changes, I think they will do better. Unfortunately, I'm not sure how to effect this.

I am an overseas student. I feel that I need more "peer support" or better relationships. After class everybody left, we never had a chance to talk. We could have more informal meetings or special occasions to develop our relationships.

I might add that I work full-time and have very little time for informal socializing with my peers. I've maintained a very narrow focus while in school—which has allowed me to progress quickly in the program, but at the expense of networking or informal interaction.

As a part of a new program, I have been experiencing what is more than usual frustration. Many procedures are being formulated as we, the first class, announce our readiness to proceed to the next step. Faculty want to help but workload scheduling relief and a PhD "mind-set" are not yet a part of the milieu. As a result, few faculty are available for more than a quick consultation. Meaningful feedback, other than on graded work, is hard to find. There is also a perception on my part that our school will do things fairly rigidly and in accord with overall nursing tradition rather than understanding or uncovering essentials and discarding those traditions without reasons behind them. I find it is like "I suffered and so you must, too."

Students learn on their own for the most part, but faculty are usually available. The course workload is manageable but we never get caught up on the readings for the courses because of the volume of material we have available to us. We all want to know it all and are frustrated at being unable to read everything and be able to discuss it. Class size is small if only doctoral students take the classes, but some courses are taken with master's students also. It is easy to see the difference in processing of the master and the PhD students. MS students think pretty superficially. PhD students are often hostile, and competitive generally. Experiences with the faculty offset the awful experiences of interacting with some of the students, especially the ones whose attitude is that because they are in a PhD program they are "special" or "superior" to everyone else. (It is one thing to think it but quite another to actually say it.) Some actually say such things as "I'm brilliant," "I was always a thinker and know I'm probably the best in the class," or some such nonsense. So, I like to interact minimally and that keeps my morale high and allows me to not roll my eyes and say "oh, brother" too often.

I have found during my doctoral program that there has been too much emphasis on research and not enough on connecting the research to the practical application needed for practice. Colleges place faculty in the tenuous position of having to produce, leaving them little time to spend mentoring students. Although I have learned a great deal from my courses I have often been frustrated with the inflexible attitudes of both my professors and my peers. Do they not understand that there is more than one way to get from point A to point B especially at this level? Do they not know that the only way knowledge grows is to pass it around? I find the level of competition between students both unacceptable and unprofessional. After all, as PhD students in nursing we are already the people to be helping other nurses grow both in understanding and professionalism and I for one am definitely not competing with them or anyone.

There is no "quality control" in many programs. It's often an implicit (and true) assumption that you'll get no less than an A in a doctoral nursing course. Very few faculty give grades based on what students actually have earned. I've seen a good deal of students doing papers or take home tests for other students. I've observed it on the fringes. Again, a quality control problem. In my instance I had an extremely supportive colleague going through school at the same time I was. My more positive experiences with course work, exams and proposal meetings are in strong contrast with some of my other colleagues. I attribute this primarily to the presence of this co-supportive colleague.

Doctoral education is a very lonely, isolated and solitary experience, especially toward the dissertation. The isolation at times is almost unbearable, but no one but you can do the thinking and the work.

I am an older graduate student and am doing my doctoral studies on a part-time basis, both of which I believe are more common to the cadre of graduate students than not. Perhaps, because I cannot be fully immersed in the academic atmosphere, I have been disappointed in a failure to sense the professional collegiality I had expected at this level of study. Somehow, I had the notion that along with research skill building, there would be opportunity for the sharing, discussion, challenging, and development of a full range of ideas and perspectives. I have been saddened to find classes are far more traditional, with papers, projects, presentations with compacted deadlines which curtail really meaningful contemplation and assimilation of new or reconfigured knowledge. Like the rest of our approach to nursing education, doctoral study seems to me the same old task orientation. Too bad we can't switch the nursing educational paradigm to truly focus on meaningful thought. But, I'll trudge along with the eternal hope that maybe after the doctoral degree will come the time for creativity and wisdom!

The transition from a master's to doctoral level was difficult. Peer relationships were much more competitive and much less supportive, however, faculty relationships improved.

The message from the students seems clear—not enough support is currently available in doctoral programs to help students succeed without major frustration. Another message is that we continue to be traditional and task oriented—even at this advanced level. Are we discouraging inquiring minds and trying to fit doctoral students into preexisting paradigms? It seems stifling and rigid from the student perspective in many cases. This can't continue.

NURSES NEED NURSES

How do we, then, improve the nursing network for our students and colleagues, and ourselves? Hamilton (1981) noted that "many professionals have strong informal networks for information sharing, guidance, and intraprofessional protection" (p. 12). Nursing could greatly benefit from high level networking circles. Administratively, colleagues can discuss how nursing can climb the mountains of managed care contracts. Educators can break the traditional patterns in the classroom, replace the rigidity with flexible new age curricula, and rid the loneliness for the student. Researchers can continue to focus on practice based research. The students have voiced concern over quality control, and fierce competition. These are also issues that need to be addressed. But if we were to try to form circles of networking nurses—arenas of sharing, guiding and professional protection, then, what steps would we take?

TAKE CARE OF OUR YOUNG

Faculty, mentors and those who teach doctoral students should teach how to succeed and how to network. Networking guidelines have been set forth by Robinson (1995). The author suggests:

1. Keep records (names, addresses, and phone numbers).
2. Attend presentations by those who are resource persons.

3. Introduce yourself to the individual and follow up with a call or letter.
4. Exchange business cards (they should be on white or off-white good quality paper).
5. Develop and focus upon your goals.
6. Be assertive—don't wait to be discovered.
7. Recognize opportunities (pp. 261–274).

Other suggestions we see as important include:

1. Communicate by Internet if possible—get E mail addresses, become familiar with the worldwide web, web servers and methods to assist you to streamline "information" contacts.
2. Join professional organizations or specialty groups.
3. Volunteer for offices that will keep you networking with nurses with similar interests.
4. Get your name on mailing lists—this automatically happens if you join nurse groups.
5. Be active in your alumnae associations. Many doctoral programs have active alumnae groups that annually meet, offer research seminars, and provide ways to continue to network and share scholarly interests.
6. Learn how to seek funding or grants that support your research or professional interests as well as individuals who can help you get funded.
7. Keep a business sense—professionals are not necessarily interested in your personal life or views.

SUMMARY

Graduates, students and nurses need to network to find support for projects and professional interests. In the business world this is done every day. It is not elaborate but is planned and well-executed. Recently, the CEO of a large metropolitan hospital noted that in his profession, and with all the job uncertainty, many executives speak daily on the phone about prospects in the industry and open job markets. This informal networking, he said, occurs throughout the country. High level managers continue each day to position themselves with those who have similar interests and job responsibilities. If needed they "work the network" to select or enhance one's career path. What these executives have learned in the words of Robinson (1995) is "utilize contacts for information and advice." Always have inroads and connections and advice about issues you are facing. Network. If nursing could informally network as the largest group of health care professionals think of all the possibilities—sharing, guiding, protecting.

Keep special people entering your lives. Chance and opportunity will then continue to knock at your door.

References

Hamilton, M. S. (1981). Mentorhood: A key to nursing leadership. *Nursing Leadership,* 4(1), 4–13.

Robinson, C. A. (1995). Networking Strategies. In Vestal, K. W. *Nursing Management—Concepts and Issues,* 2nd Edition, Philadelphia: J. B. Lippincott Co.

CHAPTER SIX

On Research

INTRODUCTION

THIS CHAPTER HAS two goals: one is to familiarize the reader with the process of writing a dissertation, and the second is to analyze trends in completed nursing dissertations. Many programs are philosophically similar in their beliefs about the steps in the dissertation process. For example, comprehensive examinations prior to candidacy, traditions such as sponsorship, and committee selection are important components and will be discussed based on review of doctoral nursing program catalogues. Student views on research assistantships will also be included, ending with a discussion on post doctoral studies. Finally, trends in doctoral research, specifically, substantive knowledge are analyzed. This later analysis was derived from review of over 900 titles of dissertations from 1990–1994.

THE DISSERTATION PROCESS

Comprehensive Examinations

The tradition of requiring an exam or "comp," that in essence validates prior knowledge of an area of nursing is a rigorous but expected requirement. Comprehensive examinations are often required during the semester the student completes formal nursing course work. In many programs two prerequisites exist prior to taking this exam; completion of a language requirement and major course work in nursing.

The "comp" assesses the student's knowledge of the discipline in nursing, the cognate and research. The examination may be written or oral or both and consist of several parts (i.e., clinical, professional, or curricular issues). This examination is often graded on a pass/fail basis with all parts successfully documented. Often, students are given two chances to complete the examination. Some programs, however, are quite stringent and require successful achievement on the first attempt.

A five-year window period is usually allowed between satisfactory completion of the exam and the final oral examination or doctoral defense. After students pass the comprehensive exam they progress to candidacy.

Candidacy

Admission to candidacy means that students are qualified to perform nursing research at a level needed for the doctoral dissertation. A GPA of 3.0 is the minimum grade average needed at this point in the process. Many programs require approval of the research proposal from the dissertation committee at this time.

Dissertation Committee

The dissertation committee often consists of four or more advisors. The members are selected by the student based upon faculty expertise and the student's ability to personally work with the faculty. This is often totally the student's choice.

The dissertation sponsor may be a faculty advisor that the student has worked with from the beginning of the doctoral program. In other cases the sponsor is a mentor that has similar research interests and/or can help develop the student's line of inquiry because of their expertise in methodology (i.e., historical analysis, phenomenology, inferential techniques).

One of the four faculty may be an "out of department" member which allows for varied expertise and perspective. For example, a statistician from a psychometric or measurement department may serve as a committee member. Having a nonnurse faculty on one's dissertation committee adds a different dimension and can strengthen dissertation development.

Dissertation

The dissertation is a substantial investigation that demonstrates competency in research, inquiry, and critical analysis. The dissertation must improve our professional knowledge base and theory development. It is an original thesis that uses empirical evidence, reflects independent thought and mastery of research techniques.

> The dissertation should constitute a contribution to knowledge. Such contributions may be the discovery of new facts, the establishment of new relations among facts already known, the solution of a problem hitherto unresolved, the formation of a new or improved method or the development of a new improved technique, the construction of a theory involving new principles, a critical study correcting errors, or establishing negatives (The Catholic University of America Catalogue, 1992–94, p. 48).

A major concern of leaders in the profession is the lack of clinically based research and scholarship in practice (Emden & Young, 1987; McClure, 1981; Miller, 1985; Stevenson, 1988). A strong goal currently in most doctoral programs is to facilitate clinical research in order to advance the practice of the profession. Past practice and perusal of lists of nurses completing dissertations have shifted from non-clinical to clinical foci—the direction is slow but changing. (See Appendix A for a topical listing of dissertations from 1990 to 1994). Students may not be encouraged to conduct clinical studies because the faculty committee may not be comfortable with this idea. Where does that leave the student? Where does it leave the profession? How then does the student succeed?

In many programs a series of dissertation seminars are designed to guide students through the process of proposal to completion of the study. A proposal is a formal outline or blueprint of the study. Students are often given the opportunity to critique each other's research proposal in small group seminars and offer suggestions to strengthen each other's study.

Faculty dissertation advisement is required. Usually a minimum of two to three semesters of full-time work is mandated. An approved dissertation proposal is submitted within two years of enrollment in the dissertation seminar.

An oral defense of the dissertation is often called "the final examination." It is a means of justifying before an advisory committee research ability and significance in building nursing knowledge. The student must follow the university format guidelines for final submission of the dissertation—a process that is quite rigorous in terms of detail and personal dedication as can be verified from the narrative comments of doctoral students:

> Students are often disheartened by the political games that are played in doctoral education. These include not giving the same information to all students within class settings or giving different responses to the student in an informal setting which change in a formal setting. An example might be agreeing to do something with a student's dissertation proposal (informally with the student) and then denying or changing the agreement when the dissertation committee convenes.

> The rigor of research and the dissertation process is a major factor in knowledge gained—this is, in fact, the focus of the dissertation.

> The most efficient way to negotiate my program's requirement is to link the candidacy paper, related field papers (answering three questions) and the dissertation proposal. The process is extremely unstructured and some of the guidelines are acquired informally from other students. I wish this was a little tighter (the linkage for the process, not the content) and emphasized earlier in the program so students are not left with three disjointed areas of study. Otherwise, growth (personal and professional) is phenomenal (with an obligatory touch of anxiety).

> Dissertation research and the content of master's and doctoral programs must build on the extension of nursing theories and the testing and development of mid-range nursing theories.

Seminars devoted to dissertation development were extremely valuable.

All course work should lead to expertise in content area (i.e., the identification of researchable questions, state of the art in nursing knowledge in an area of practice). Dissertation quality should be consistent across areas of specialization. Students would receive recognition of contributions made to faculty and research efforts. Nursing research should address patient issues not nurse (i.e., attitudes, learning styles) characteristics.

One major, unresolved frustration at this point in time, is the aloneness of the dissertation process. Faculty and peers attempt to be supportive but this is only somewhat helpful. Although I entered this program to learn how to do research (and this has been a major component of the program), the opportunity to develop my critical thinking skills has been an unexpected dividend!

I think retelling of "war stories" helps to perpetuate the myth that only survivors get the dissertation finished without a major life crisis. I would like to see a more positive approach—don't nurses already know that our goals are not easy? By the way, a supportive committee really makes the process go smoother.

SELECTING AN AREA OF STUDY

Prior to selecting an area of study doctoral students develop an appreciation of the trilogy—*theory, research,* and *practice.* Students learn that nursing theory is purposeful and that leaders have demonstrated areas of "convergence" over the last 30 years. As highlighted by Jennings (1987) the profession values the need for *theory,* recognizes the components of theory, accepts the domain concepts, and identifies that "multiple modes" of theory are needed in gaining a better understanding of theory (p. 64). Differing opinions also exist on semantics, labels and a need to better connect theory and practice. The need for doctoral students to evaluate nursing theory beyond structured guidelines for critique as done on the master's level exists. Using a mature comparative view of the differing paradigms of science occurs on the doctoral level. Doctoral students use nursing theory as a format for future research, design unique theory or test current paradigms in their research agendas (Lutjens & Horan, 1992). According to doctoral students:

> The content areas of nursing administration/systems (which is my content area) in my school did not take enough advantage of the theoretical and empirical works from organizational psychology, management, and business disciplines. We read only from the nursing literature which is too restrictive and immature. Nursing administration/systems programs need to learn from these disciplines! There is nothing wrong with this. Then nursing management research won't get published using Herzberg's theory, which the organizational behaviors discipline discarded 20 years ago. As a profession we look out of touch with the cutting edge of knowledge development. Finally, the nursing data base CINAHL needs to be integrated with the mainstream of social science data bases. There is a saying "nurses read everyone else's literature, but no one reads ours." No wonder, they can't access it! I don't imply by this that nursing doesn't have a unique disciplinary area or that nursing needs the acceptance of other disciplines to be legitimate. I only suggest integrating and exposing nursing literature to a wider audience. For example, some social psychologist might be interested in how nursing has used empathy in practice or theoretical development. I'm sure that many other disciplines would benefit from nursing citations in their review of the literature on selected topics.

> I am in a BSN to PhD program—after completing all course work (72 + hours post BSN), I remain "unqualified" to teach in nursing—transcripts are not submissible, and only an MSN certifies an individual to teach. I find this frustrating as my research and dissertation will entail approximately two more years of time. Until then I must remain in practice at a BSN level. Other disciplines (as usual) do not operate under the rigidity that nursing does. Interestingly, my program has done a marvelous job expanding my horizons and my perspectives. It's very strong in philosophy and research. Now that I see the possibilities and options, I must continue to succumb to the realm of traditional nursing, though—frustrating! Nursing must become open to other strategies, options. Perhaps our primary hope lies in doctorally educated nurses (PhD) who have also seen the pos-

sibilities. It has been my experience that emphasis remains on quantitative research. This is unacceptable. My hope is that qualitative research becomes as valued as quantitative.

I believe the strength of my doctoral program has been the depth of research methods course work available in seminar format. These were all conducted by nursing faculty and complemented the year of graduate statistics courses I took in the biostatistics department. Nurse scientists are in a unique position to provide leadership in health care research. They bring clinical expertise and science into arenas which previously have seen those backgrounds in separate disciplines, i.e., medicine and statistics.

Nursing needs to standardize the curricula and expectations of the EdD vs. DNS vs. PhD. There is too much confusion. Schools without significant research activity ongoing should not have doctoral programs. Too many of our programs prepare inferior researchers. Research courses should emphasize practical projects; students should be exposed to and allowed to participate in ongoing research studies so that they learn the practical skills (such as computer data analysis) needed to conduct research.

Doctoral education is a research degree. Although exposure to literature in a variety of areas may impact my clinical practice, my first goal in obtaining this degree was not to become an expert clinician. You raise some interesting questions as to whether the doctoral degree is designed to prepare nurses as educators or administrators. I believe some of the course work here offers emphasis in those areas, but there is no requirement for these components. Exposure to a variety of educational techniques might be useful, but seems to be a focus of a different degree. My preparation is geared to help me examine ways of answering questions that pertain to nursing and allow for the expansion of nursing knowledge through research.

The PhD is intended to be the highest terminal degree in any field. Doctoral education should reflect this distinction in the content of each type of doctoral program. The content of a PhD program in nursing science should be directed to the extant theory base of nursing, i.e., those theories that are unique to nursing, like Roy, Rogers, Orem, and Parse. The process of doctoral education in nursing should be directed toward expanding this theory base. This is the only scenario that is consistent with the pattern of doctoral education in any other field. The continuing practices of borrowing theories from medicine, physiology, pharmacology, psychology, and sociology—calling the work "nursing" only because a nurse is doing it—must change or higher education in nursing is doomed to second-class status and eventual obscurity. One of the major problems in nursing education is the lack of attention to nursing's own theory base. Another, at the master's and doctoral levels, is the inequity between quantitative and qualitative methods. The future of nursing is in the expansion of our theory base as an emergent human science. This should be the overriding primary concern of doctoral education in nursing.

Our program has a strong quantitative focus, however, several experienced doctoral faculty with funded projects of qualitative research have allowed me to get a balance. It was only through independent study, however, and not an integral part of the curriculum. I have been fortunate in having positive mentoring experiences, although many of my peers have not.

The PhD nursing program in which I am currently enrolled is excellent. There is a very strong emphasis on research and there is preparation and acceptance and support for both quantitative and/or qualitative methodologies.

The doctoral education I have received has been quite outstanding. Research has been a key focus, but there has been an exceptional blending of other roles which link with research. These include: practice, executive roles, public policy, education and epistemologic expansion in nursing science.

The doctoral program is clearly the place for sophisticated research behaviors.

Students in doctoral programs are not arriving there as complete research neophytes.

Nursing science will only advance through systematic inquiry.

It is more important to instill a true spirit of inquiry (with which one appreciates all one does) than to focus on specific research or statistics skills.

Research that is done poorly is worse than not doing research.

I am disillusioned with doctoral research with so many flaws in design, data collection, etc.

Total immersion in research is inappropriate for nursing and more focus should be on policy, politics and more innovative practice.

Nursing *research* is the "systematic inquiry into problems associated with illness, health, and care" (Gortner, 1980, p. 180). Practice-based research has been identified as a critical need (McClure, 1981). Doctoral students nationwide are aware of this need.

Areas of nursing knowledge have been clearly defined as a discipline: clinical knowledge, conceptual knowledge and empirical knowledge (Schultz & Meleis, 1988). A group of strategies to enhance further knowledge development have been proposed (Stevenson, 1988). Stevenson viewed the need for nurses to promote research and knowledge development on a broader scale, i.e., investigating the entire family unit or community as they interact with the environment, yet not losing site of the study of humans, holistically. Voids in nursing research are identified. They include: fundamental knowledge for nurses to research nursing therapeutic approaches in basic areas such as decubiti, immobility, confusion, pain, restlessness, and fatigue; research to improve nursing practice and clinical nursing implementations; health and wellness; and family research, whereby the entire family is investigated; and cross-cultural research. From the student:

I feel what is missing in my doctoral education is a course on grant writing and research proposals. Also, at our university nurse educators are so busy with their own research that it is quite difficult to find an advisor or even to get appointments to see them.

Students in doctoral education should select research that improves nursing care and patient health.

Doctoral programs should prepare nurses to pursue interdisciplinary research as a primary investigator.

Schools without significant research activity ongoing should not have doctoral programs—too many of our programs prepare inferior researchers.

Research has to be brought out of the lab and into the lives of the students, as something interesting that they can use to gain control over their lives.

I have learned more about research and making an impact on health and health care services, by working in a multi-disciplinary center at the university than I ever did in all my other 15 plus doctoral courses.

Courses related to research were abstract and disconnected from the real world.

Once I finished my course work and was doing my research there were no formal arenas for me to meet with other students to discuss issues, to get or to offer support.

McClure (1981) addressed two critical factors that affect *practice*-based research. The first is the lack of commitment to research for nursing in the practice area and the second is the lack of interest among nurse researchers to study practice problems (p. 67). Miller (1985) sought to "alleviate the schizophrenia afflicting nursing" by recombining theory and practice. Miller suggested that ideally the theory-practice gap could be bridged by nurse practitioners but that this is not likely. She suggested that faculty joint appointments would be a step in the direction of "reintegration of theory and practice" (p. 423).

Nursing research must drive our clinical practice. Doctoral students appreciate theory and practice connections. They want to bring research into the practice setting using innovative approaches. The spirit of inquiry has been fostered at the doctoral level. Students encourage interdisciplinary research and global perspectives that focus on policy and politics affecting our practice.

I have the pleasure of being with fellow students from a variety of practice backgrounds including strong clinical practice and education. Doctoral education is moving more and more away from faculty needs and into practice—that's where the theory-research-practice circle will be accomplished.

In nursing, I feel we need to do a better job at accepting, even welcoming, diversity. In order to move forward as a profession, we need to become strong on many fronts—education, administration, clinical practice and research. The personal characteristics and makeup of an expert educator may be different from those of a researcher, for example. Those who are excellent teachers of clinical practice may not be the same people who can pull in RO1 grants—but a strong school should be composed of both. Likewise, those who work in the service setting should be able to have a research component to their jobs, and have workloads which can accommodate research. In my perception, medicine has done a much better job at encouraging and accommodating a triple focus of education, clinical practice and research for each physician, than we do in nursing—we seem to have to pick one.

Since beginning doctoral education, I feel I am gaining new skills and knowledge, but without clinical practice I am losing clinical skills and experiences. With the constant change in clinical practice, it is very easy to lose touch . . . research must come from clinical practice. Without my time as a research associate I would not be in the hospital at all. I've seen more researchers who have no idea what actually happens with patients—the demand of research and teaching roles overwhelms the clinician role. This leads to research findings that aren't valued or utilized by practitioners.

My program places equal emphasis on theory development, knowledge structuring and research at present. There are no formal mechanisms for linking doctoral students to the practice setting. This is a major shortcoming in my view. The issues that will improve collaboration among researchers, educators, and practitioners are centered in the clinical setting. Doctorally prepared nurses have the knowledge necessary to advance nursing theory but to be truly relevant to the care of patients and families, nursing questions should be evolving from collaborations with clinicians. Whether theory drives research or research drives theory is not the critical issue for nursing. The quality of the research questions and their relationship to patient care are important issues to me.

I very strongly believe that more doctorally prepared nurses are needed in clinical settings. Many administrators hold the opinion that the terminal degree in the hospital (and other direct-care arenas) is a master's degree. As a clinician seeking a PhD, I have encountered no faculty that disagree with my stance, but I have certainly been a minority—most fellow students are faculty, or unemployed with plans to seek faculty positions. I further disagree with the position that substantive research can be conducted only by those in faculty positions. I realize that the support and expertise available in a university setting are important to effect such projects, and especially for funding, but it is important to recognize that clinical practice settings provide an endless array of questions and research opportunities.

We need to encourage nurses at all levels of education to continue to learn and to be responsible for instituting change in their environment. Research has to be brought out of the lab and into the lives of the students, as something interesting that they can use to gain control over their lives.

Doctoral programs should prepare nurses to pursue interdisciplinary research as a primary investigator if the area of interest is research. All areas (research, education and administration) should prepare the nurse to manage! A mini-MBA course to manage educational money or research funding will allow nurses to manage their money and time, and allow a balance of their time to their area of interest. When will nursing acknowledge that without specific knowledge, advancement for many clinical nurses is bound to fail? Nurses should be more grounded in quantitative statistics if only to aid in management or to counter those who feel qualitative research is too soft.

Research must come from our clinical practice.

I have seen nurse researchers who have no idea what actually happens with patients.

There needs to be greater acceptance of doctorally prepared nurses at the bedside working to improve care of clients.

Research efforts should focus on solving clinical dilemmas pertinent to the client.

There is too much emphasis on research and not enough on connecting the research to the practical applications needed for practice.

My practice is clinical with a research base. My dissertation will be clinical as well. My research component has been presented in a very structured way throughout the program and I feel that I have gained valuable knowledge.

The need to tighten the connection between theory, research, and practice are continual challenges for the doctoral student. They are challenges that are recognized and being addressed. Themes that have emerged in the student data include a strong need to focus on practice-based research and the need to allow the student to do so in the academic setting. The quality of the research is of sincere concern with equitable distribution of both quantitative and qualitative methods of research.

RESEARCH ASSISTANTS

The doctoral education process affords an opportunity for students to work with faculty on research in an assistant capacity. Students are given credit on their transcripts or earn money for participating in research endeavors. Students learn the research process, tutor other students and develop teaching skills if they are involved in the classroom or lab setting. As participants noted:

> The best part of my doctoral education has been being able to go to school full-time, as well as being a research assistant for one of my professors. This "immersion" into academia has been most worthwhile and has really shaped my experience as a "doctoral student." I realize that it is not always possible for all students to go to school full time or be RAs but this avenue should be emphasized to all! My RA position has allowed me to be involved with many research projects and has facilitated learning nursing research "hands on."

> Research assistantship is an excellent way to gain experience and a few extra dollars while in school.

> What I think was very helpful in my doctoral education, which I think should be available to all doctoral education in general, is faculty mentorship and having research experience either as a graduate student, research assistant or just working in the faculty's lab.

> Working as a research assistant enhances the student's ability to design and implement a research project/dissertation.

> Experience as a research assistant on an established research team has been invaluable.

I have a research assistantship and no outside employment. I am enjoying studying using the library and the computer. I have sufficient time to become immersed in studies most of the time. I think research methodology and statistics courses are fascinating. I think learning to use the mainframe with SPSS and SAS for statistical analysis is crucial for a PhD in nursing. I think nurse researchers should be able to do their own data analysis.

Emphasize practical projects. Students should be exposed to and allowed to participate in ongoing research studies so that they learn the practical skills such as computer data analysis.

I have had the opportunity to have a research assistantship for two years. This has been a wonderful learning experience. It has reinforced my course work especially in the area of research methodology.

I have been fortunate to work as a research assistant in a very large, federally funded nursing study for almost two years. This has afforded me invaluable experience in all facets of nursing research. Those who do not have this opportunity are missing a great deal.

The assistant role encourages collaborative efforts of faculty and students outside the classroom. It promotes dialogue on research projects, is stimulating and gives the student a "hands on" view of the research process. It can be an apprenticeship for future research. Assistants are often given recognition for their student contributions which further promotes professionalism and mutual collaboration.

POST-DOCTORAL WORK

Research doesn't end with the completion of a dissertation. In fact, many say it is just a beginning. Post-doctoral nurse fellows date back to 1955. Fellowships include a research project with merit, a sponsor and/or cosponsor who are dedicated to the project, resources, and a time commitment of two or more years (Hinshaw & Lucas, 1993).

The opportunity to fine tune research skills in a concentrated area and develop one's research career are afforded in a post-doctoral fellowship. It is a true dedication, in that both career and financial sacrifices are made in pursuit of their goal. The contribution of excellence for the sake of nursing science is quite compelling. Williams (1988) cited three reasons that the discipline of nursing is particularly ready for post-doctoral study: (1) We now have a "meaningful number" of doctoral graduates, (2) increased levels of support exist and (3) the "complexity and demands" of clinically based research are present and need to be addressed.

The National Institutes of Health, The National Center for Nursing Research, American Nurses Association Registered Nurse Fellowship and Clinical Fellowship Programs for Ethnic/Racial Minorities and the Kellogg Foundation are all funding agencies for nursing research. Lev, Souder, and Topp highlight funding sources in the spring issue of *Image* (1990). Specific awards available to nurse researchers from these agencies may include the National Research Service Award Post-doctoral Fellowship, Robert Wood Johnson Clinical Nurse Scholars Program, Academic Investigator award and awards for clinically trained nurses or junior faculty members who are recent doctoral graduates. Post-doctoral fellowships are available in many clinical areas such as psychosocial oncology and gerontology.

Nursing doctoral students throughout the country were asked about plans for post-doctoral study in the distant future. Few had knowledge about the "postdoc" concept and one participant stated that post-doctoral work was not encouraged. One wonders how much emphasis, particularly in research classes is placed on the tradition of the post-doctoral work. Others feel post-doctoral work is limited and not realistic: "Expecting all students to pursue a postdoc is crazy. The number of postdocs available are limited. Also, it does not take into account the realities of women's lives. It is difficult to pick up and go with my children and husband while he makes the majority of the family income."

Perhaps there is a giant gap in our current doctoral education if we are unable to develop systematic programs of research that contribute to nursing science. Attention to all aspects of the research experience should be a priority for faculty leaders. Assisting the student to select an area of study, understand the trilogy of theory, research and practice connections and internalize methods for "succeeding" in the dissertation process are key issues.

DOCTORAL DISSERTATIONS:
TOPICS OVER THE LAST DECADE

In 1988, Williams questioned the amount of "clinical research" occurring in doctoral programs as well as the qualified mentors to guide students in clinical research. Contemporary content in doctoral dissertations may be more educational in origin because of time constraints and perhaps due to the lack of faculty with active ongoing research. This was in essence validated by Wiley (1989) in a study of deans and directors of doctoral programs who were queried about dissertation topics accepted in their PhD programs. The majority responded that they accepted doctoral dissertations that focused on nursing administration and nursing education in addition to clinical nursing. Dissertation topics were often accepted if they fit the mentor's expertise and past experience in research.

It may be a matter of logistics that impacts on the amount of clinical research being generated among nurse doctorates. However, if we are to generate knowledge about health and understanding human illness our research must be clinical and practice-based in the future.

The good news is that the literature reveals a substantial effort to concentrate our effort in clinical nursing research. Loomis (1985) analyzed the content of 319 dissertations from 1976–1982. The author found that 78.4 percent of the dissertations pertained to clinical nursing and 21.6 percent to social issues in nursing. Clinical nursing research dissertations were defined as *actual/potential health problems* (developmental life changes, acute health deviations, chronic health deviations, and stressors), *human response systems* (physical, emotional, cognitive, family and social), and *clinical decision making* (data collection, diagnosis, planning, treatment and evaluation). Social issues included profession/policy, social decision making and specific units of analysis such as individual group or organization. The author noted that 18 of 20 doctoral programs were weighted with a clinical focus and seven programs only focused on clinical dissertations. The author concluded that clinical research within nursing doctoral programs was a trend over the six-year studies.

Sherwin, Bevil, Adler and Watson (1993) surveyed 434 deans

and directors of baccalaureate and higher degree programs about current and future need, contribution and funding capability of researchers prepared within five areas: psychosocial processes, biophysical processes, health care delivery systems and administration, education, and methodology and instrumentation. Deans confirmed that the majority of nursing research activities is currently on phenomena in the psychosocial or behavioral domain. The deans noted that future funding would be highest for nursing inquiry into the biophysical phenomena, yet viewed this type of research as less necessary than behavioral research. Deans viewed delivery systems and administration more favorably than education in terms of future contribution to nursing theory and funding. Educational research was perceived as having the poorest chance of receiving funding and viewed as the least important to nursing.

Meleis (1992) discussed strategies for doctoral students to develop scholarship. Also noted was that research courses and those dealing with theory and statistics are different than "fields of interest" in nursing. Students cannot perform research in isolation of the substantive fields in nursing such as health promotion, coping with transitions, environment, primary health care, cardiovascular rehabilitation and the developmental field of pediatric nursing.

So then, what are the current topical trends of nursing dissertations? We reviewed over 900 titles published over five years by Sigma Theta Tau (1990–1994) of "recent nursing doctorates." It is evident that nursing doctoral programs are developing scholarship in the substantive fields (see Appendix A). Ten trends were noted in this research including a shift to more clinical foci and clinical nursing research such as pulmonary and cardiac clinical nursing implementation. Many studies are still being reported from the education and administrative perspective—over 200 studies—the largest of the ten areas. A summary of these ten trends follows:

1. Women's issues—172 studies
2. Transitions in the elderly—103 studies
3. Cardiac rehab and cardiovascular nursing—65 studies
4. Pediatric and developmental variables—152 studies

5. HIV/AIDS—21 studies
6. Pulmonary and oxygenation—13 studies
7. Medical Surgical knowledge—79 studies
8. Oncology nursing—40 studies
9. Psychiatric/psychosocial knowledge—47 studies
10. Nursing education/administration—212 studies

We concur with the writings of Meleis and note that nursing research has shifted to substantive areas in nursing. We also concur with the earlier findings of Loomis who identified a trend toward clinical research in the abstracts and titles surveyed from the period of 1976–1982.

Omissions are essential to address as well. The omissions in nursing doctoral research reported by Loomis (1985) included cultural/environmental stressors, family, social and cultural human response systems, planning treatment and evaluation in clinical decision making, and the areas of economics, history, and politics. Many of these gaps are less evident in doctoral dissertations today. From a cultural perspective global studies on women in Botswana, Greek Canadian widows, Hispanic and Mexican Americans and the pluralistic health care system of Taiwan, for example, add to our nursing knowledge. The dissertations reviewed included cultural and environmental stressors particularly within the categories of women's issues and cardiac nursing research for example. Social issues such as economics and politics are better developed in the body of administrative literature of nurse doctorates receiving their degrees in the past five-to-six years. For example, studies on nursing resource consumption, utilization and outcomes of home health care, work design and cost of patient care are evident.

SUMMARY

Research at the doctoral level is leaning toward a clinical focus, thus contributing to nursing's substantive body of knowledge. This is an important trend if the profession is to continue to grow and verify information unique to the profession. This chapter expands on the brief discussion related to research in Chapter 3 and provides further evidence of the focus on quantitative rather than qualitative research in nursing. Appendix A adds to the discussion by providing a listing by topic of the dissertations completed in the last four years, and highlighting the areas of focus.

References

Bessent, H. (1989). Post-doctoral leadership training for women of color. *Journal of Professional Nursing, 5*(5), 279–282.

Boston College Graduate Catalog (1992–1993).

Catholic University of America School of Nursing Catalogue (1992–1994). pp. 45–49.

Emden, C., & Young, W. (1987). Theory development in nursing: Australian nurses advance global debate. *The Australian Journal of Advanced Nursing, 6*(3), 22–40.

Gortner, S. R. (1980). Nursing science in transition. *Nursing Research, 29*(3), 180–183.

Hinshaw, A. S., & Lucas, M. D. (1993). Post-doctoral education—a new tradition for nursing research. *Journal of Professional Nursing, 9*(6), 309.

Jennings, B. M. (1987). Nursing theory development: Successes and challenges. *Journal of Advanced Nursing, 12*, 63–69.

Lev, E., Souder, E., & Topp, R. (1990). The post-doctoral fellowship experience. *Image, 22*(2), 116–120.

Loomis, M. E. (1985). Emerging content in nursing: An analysis of dissertation abstracts and titles: 1976–1982. *Nursing Research, 43*(2), 113–119.

Lutjens, L. R., & Horan, M. L. (1992). Nursing theory in nursing education: An educational imperative. *Journal of Professional Nursing, 8*(5), 276–281.

Louisiana State University Catalog/Bulletin (1992–1994), pp. 30–31.

McClure, M. L. (1981). Promoting practice-based research: A critical need. *Journal of Nursing Administration*, 66–70.

Meleis, A. (1992). On the way to scholarship: From Master's to doctorate. *Journal of Professional Nursing, 8*(6), 328–334.

Miller, A. (1985). The relationship between nursing theory and nursing practice. *Journal of Advanced Nursing, 10,* 417–424.

Reflections (1990–1994). Recent Nursing Doctorates. Sigma Theta Tau.

Schultz, P. R., & Meleis, A. I. (1988). Nursing epistemology: Traditions, insights, questions. *Image, 20*(4), 217–221.

Sherwin, L. N., Bevil, C. A., Adler, D., & Watson, P. G. (1993). Education for the future: A national survey of nursing deans about need and demand for nurse researchers. *Journal of Professional Nursing, 9*(4), 195–203.

Stevenson, J. S. (1988). Nursing knowledge development: Into era II. *Journal of Professional Nursing, 4*(3), 152–162.

University of Alabama at Birmingham Catalog, School of Nursing (1991–1993), p. 42

University of Illinois at Chicago Graduate Catalog (1991–1993), p. 58.

University of Rochester Graduate Bulletin (1992–1994), pp. 56–57.

Widener University Graduate Bulletin (1992–1994), p. 195.

Wiley, M. (1989). Focus of research for PhD in Nursing. *Journal of Nursing Education, 28*(4), 190–192.

Williams, C. A. (1988). Career Development of the Nurse-Scientist. The new doctorate faces a post-doctoral. *Journal of Professional Nursing, 4*(2), 73.

Williams, M. (1988). Dissertation topics. *Research in Nursing & Health* (1988), 11, p. iii–iv.

CHAPTER SEVEN

On Commitment

Then said a rich man, Speak to us of Giving.
  And he answered:
You give but little when you give of your possessions.
It is when you give of yourself that you truly give.

                                        Gibran, 1951, pp. 18–22

INTRODUCTION

THE TREMENDOUS COMMITMENT shown by nurses in doctoral education is impressive. The financial burdens, long commutes, sacrificed
time with family and friends, and endless fatigue make one wonder
why nurses are so giving. The message from Gibran is clear . . .
giving freely of oneself by choice is what gives meaning to our very
existence. The absence of or lack of commitment in nursing is seen
as the inability to truly give freely and by choice of all that one has
to offer. But, where does commitment begin? Where does commitment end? Can one be over committed? Undercommitted?

This chapter will examine commitment by nurses, the nature of
commitment and its relevance for nursing, and provide as well a
thematic analysis of the concept of commitment by nurses to each
other, the profession, and self. Upon chapter completion, the reader
will have a deeper understanding of the nature of the everyday lived
experience of commitment as perceived by nurses.

COMMITMENT: TRUE MEANING

There are few literary works available which address the philosophical aspect of commitment in nursing. Levenstein (1986) noted that "One of the many things about the nursing profession that I find fascinating is that, while all professions have their array of commitments, nurses' are far more complicated and numerous" (p. 75). In addition, the author believes there is a mutual obligation in human relationships to fulfill promises made.

Nurses experience many relationships within the health care delivery system that are two way streets. Relationships in which mutual obligation is expected include those with patients, other nurses, educators, the physician, and the hospital or academic setting. Levenstein asserted:

> Unfortunately, the more numerous the commitments, the more difficult it is to implement each of them—particularly if, at any given moment they are incompatible with each other. It is at this point in her or his experience that the nurse encounters the special burdens of the profession, what the industrial psychologist calls role overload and role conflict (p. 75).

Robert K. Merton (1974) provided insight related to the phenomenon of commitment in his discussion of the tremendous pressure for loyalty and commitment exerted on employees by the institutions in which they work. Merton indicated that institutions are continually striving to harness the energies of employees to best serve the needs of the institution. Human energy possesses limits however, and the energies of each individual are allocated to many things in life. Merton (1974) stated:

> Modern man is typically enmeshed in a web of group affiliations and hence subject to the pushes and pulls of many claimant to his commitment. In modern society, the amount of time that an individual legitimately owes to his employer is normatively and even legally established; this makes it possible for him to have time for his family or other non-occupational associations (Merton, 1974, p. 2).

Merton's discussion of the many demands on human energy for commitment can be closely related to the many demands for commitment which nurses face. For example, hospital administrators demand time from nurses, college Deans demand scholarly work. Nurses have many commitments at work and have many commitments at home. At some point one's energy to remain committed is drained and something gives . . . either the nurse, her career, or her home and personal life.

Sister Madeleine Clemence (1966) made a significant contribution to the literature in nursing with her article entitled "Existentialism: A Philosophy of Commitment." Sister Clemence provides a philosophical perspective to the subject of commitment noting that commitment can mean a number of things such as a promise, or a dedication. Clemence (1966) asserted:

> In existentialism, commitment means even more: a willingness to live fully one's own life, to make that life meaningful through acceptance of, rather than detachment from, all that it may hold of both joy and sorrow (Clemence, 1966, p. 55).

Clemence (1966) noted that if the nurse is truly committed she or he will feel and become a part of everything that one faces in nursing, including the frustrations and problems. This bonding or connection will ultimately enrich the nurse, the patient, and the profession.

Tourtillot (1981) stated that commitment was intensely personal and that it was internally motivated. She further stated that when the quality of commitment exists in nurses it exists independently of their degrees or titles. The author also noted that too often we confuse commitment with dedication. She viewed dedication as more of an acceptance of the status quo. She further noted that it is much easier to reward and nurture dedication as opposed to commitment. Tourtillot asserted:

> For the committed nurse the rewards are almost nonexistent, since the committed nurse in being who she must be, necessarily stands

against stereotypes of what she is and what she does. She does not need praise from others to know the worth of her effort. Her reward is the effort. Her effort defines her worth. Indeed her effort is her reason for being. (Tourtillott, 1981, p. 2)

Quinn and Smith (1987) discuss commitment in relationship to its professional and ethical underpinnings. The authors stated that entering a profession such as nursing is a personal experience and that the experience of making this personal decision means involving oneself in a system of roles that are socially defined. The professional commitment is viewed differently as it is a public proclamation made to all potential users of a professional's services: that is, it involves persona in a way that a purely private decision usually does not. "In effect, the professional makes a promise to society" (Quinn & Smith, 1987, p. 7). According to Haughey (1975) life will be found when "a person is willing to particularize his or her choices in life and does so in such a way that he does not identify himself in terms of what he has or hopes to hold on to but in terms of who he is and who he intends to be present to" (p. 21). Haughey further noted that the underpinnings of commitment include three components. Haughey stated that every commitment involves a choice, every commitment involves a promise, and every commitment involves the problem of reconciling freedom with commitment.

Regarding Choice: "Our Choices, more than any other act or operation of our faculties individuate and define us" (Haughey, 1975, p. 22). Acts of personal choice are what shape the person. Individuals do not grow upward physically, outward spatially, or inward reflectively, but by choosing according to Haughey.

Regarding Promise: "The simple act of promising has something to teach us about commitment. The promise is a particular kind of choice. Every commitment involves a promise. The most formal promises we make are commitments. The one making a promise is expressing his faith in his own power to do what he wills to do. One gives his word because he is free to do so and does so freely" (Haughey, 1975, pp. 27–28).

Regarding Freedom: Therefore one makes a promise when one

commits oneself to someone or something and that promise is made freely. Given this notion of freedom Haughey emphasized that understanding of the relationship between freedom and commitment is imperative.

Haughey (1975) maintained that refusal to make commitments and unfaithfulness in keeping commitments that have been made are usually the consequence of the notion of freedom. According to Haughey it would seem that freedom and commitment are incompatible given the notion that the more commitments you have the less free you will be. The author also asserted that no one's freedom exists apart from a particular context, and that it is only in the exercise of one's freedom that one assures it; by nonexercise one runs the risk of losing it. One can apply the underpinnings expressed by the author to nursing . . . the decision to first enter the profession, remain in it, and seek professional education on the baccalaureate, master, and then doctoral level ultimately has its foundation in the phenomenon of commitment.

Doctoral students make a personal choice in seeking this degree and may encounter some hardship along the way. One student asserted:

> The greatest problem I face is one of timing and expectations—most of the PhD students I know are employed—many in academia. Doctoral course work is not offered at times conducive to employment. Nevertheless, the PhD program faculty expect full commitment to doctoral work while my own employer (university) expects my full commitment. Whereas my own dean (employer) has been supportive and helpful, I find academic work draws greatly on my creativity and critical thought thereby draining "thinking time" to truly synthesize my doctoral studies away from those studies. I miss the long, cathartic opportunities to assimilate and create meaning that I had in my master's program. At that time I worked as a staff nurse and I could leave that at the hospital. My first priority was education, followed by employment. Now, employed in academia, I find my priorities reversed and feel great frustration at all the ideas and thoughts that are never fully developed because it's time to move on to the next quarter and all my contemplative time has been used.

EXPRESSIONS OF COMMITMENT

Rinaldi Carpenter (1989) examined the phenomenon of commitment as an existential and humanistic experience. She captured the phenomenon of commitment within the lifeworld of nurses through interviewing nurses and requesting verbal description of personal experiences of commitment. The resultant linguistic transformation (van Manen, 1984) allowed the nursing community to grasp the nature and significance of the experience of commitment in a way not previously viewed. Seven thematic elements were identified by the author that richly portrayed why nurses, as professionals, commit.

Altruism

When one is perceived to be committed to something, one dedicates their life to the particular cause to which they are committed. With this commitment comes sacrifice, and an obligation to that which you are committed. The unselfish regard for and devotion to the welfare of others manifest themselves daily. There is an obligation to never give up or stop fighting for the particular cause to which one is committed. This obligation is not only an obligation to yourself, but also to those individuals whose lives may be affected. Personal sacrifice and altruism, as components of the experience of commitment, occur on many different levels and in many different areas of life.

Devotion

When one is experiencing commitment, one is experiencing a devotion to someone or something. There is a strong, emotional response to whatever it is that one is committed to and a belief that what you are doing is right. The center of attention becomes the activity to which one is devoting oneself. When you commit you make a promise both to yourself and others to do the best that you can. This involves accuracy, hard work, and concentration. Investment of self, and devotion are perceived to be required.

Dedication

Dedication and commitment are perceived by nurses to mean the same thing or have similar meanings. The experience of dedication or commitment stems from enjoying those activities in which one is involved. Commitment is perceived to grow from an investment of oneself in something that is an important part of one's life.

Caring

Commitment also means caring . . . that you care enough to do your best for someone or something, and that you will not give up. Caring is an integral component of commitment. When true caring exists on the part of the nurse, the nurse is perceived to function in a responsible and accountable manner.

Trust

The characteristics of commitment and caring are perceived to be necessary if trust is to develop. Trust is an essential component of commitment. Trust is a direct offshoot of the nurses' commitment.

Loyalty

Nurses experience loyalty to many—family, colleagues, employing institution. They are also committed to the profession and to self.

These same thematic expressions of commitment apply to nurses seeking a doctoral degree. The decision to commit to an advanced (for many terminal) degree has led nurses on a path to successfully achieve this goal. Without commitment, doctoral students would not succeed. Without commitment, leaders would not emerge in the profession.

The unselfish giving that occurs as nurses sacrifice family, career, and life events in pursuit of the doctorate is notable. There is an obligation, truly to never give up or stop but to keep on going. The experience of commitment in doctoral education is altruistic.

The strong, emotional devotion by the doctoral student to complete projects in a timely manner, conduct research and participate in scholarly activities is also notable. They are devoted in spite of long commutes, sleepless nights, and a project that is always due. The experience of commitment in doctoral education encompasses devotion.

The stimulating setting, faculty, and peers make the process of doctoral education enjoyable. The constant academic rigor is challenging . . . but the benefit of broadening one's mind and awareness is awesome. The experience of commitment in doctoral education embraces dedication.

Doctoral students commit to caring. They care to be the very best and sometimes the competition is excessive. The essence, though, of this caring to be the best is focused on a belief and realization that they can effect change in the profession. The experience of commitment in doctoral education includes caring.

Doctoral students trust as a result of their caring. They "trust" that they will be given the guidance and endurance to fulfill the expectations of the degree. They trust that with a lot of hard work and confidence they can achieve. They believe that although the road may be long and tortuous it is achievable. The experience of commitment in doctoral education includes trust.

Finally, students at this level are loyal to many. As leaders they are a minority among other nurses who realize that it is up to them to propose and implement change in nursing. They continue to be loyal to many (including self) because the experience of commitment cannot be made without this loyalty. Several doctoral students in nursing expressed these thoughts:

I feel very strongly that I have grown in my profession of nursing through doctoral education. While I have some research methodology, stats, etc. in my clinical master's program, my knowledge of these has increased greatly through the doctoral program. My program is in a strong commuter university and serves a purpose by providing doctoral education in its summer programs and throughout the academic year. I have felt strongly, however, that for my own growth I needed to be in residence in order to benefit from the exposure to the faculty year-round as well as other residential students.

Up to this point in my education those degrees I have attained have very much been a validation of much of what I already knew. Pursuing my PhD has been a bit different. In addition to stretching my brain and endurance it is a personal odyssey. Truly a lived experience of finding out what I'm all about . . . a love-hate relationship. I'm sure once my dissertation is done I'll be a happy camper.

Doctoral study is extremely challenging on a cognitive level, but it really hasn't affected my over all self-confidence which was pretty good to begin with or I wouldn't have gotten this far. Now, my self-confidence in doing specific research tasks, etc. has increased, but I do not relate that to my personal level of confidence. It has challenged me. It is great to study at a school where the faculty and the students are of a high caliber. The faculty is actively involved with grants—many that are nationally funded. The only problem sometimes is getting access to them, especially when a grant is due.

My program has been grounded in nursing theory, statistical analysis and field research. Because I have continued my clinical practice I do not feel remote from the day-to-day practicalities of nursing, but I worry about that happening if I do full-time research. I also worry about the lack of preparation for teaching in my own program, although I don't know where it could be fit into the curriculum. I guess I see teaching positions as more available than positions on research teams. I wonder if I am over-educating myself for opportunities in nursing as a master's prepared clinical specialist. All this may be unrealistic anxiety. Time will tell . . . Thanks for asking for input.

The type of program is of secondary importance. The most important determinant of impact upon the professional is the strength of a nurse's identity as a nurse. Doctoral education is important for the highest levels of all nursing functions—practice, education and administration. Research is a component of all these areas. Doctoral programs should not be building self-confidence and self-esteem. Rather, they should add to and augment mature personalities who are already confident and secure in their abilities. At this level, a certain attainment of personal integration and maturity is a necessary prerequisite to academic success.

I am responsible for my commitment to excellence in the role I assume after graduation.

Rinaldi Carpenter (1989) researched "who and what the nurse is committed to" (p. 65). Through her interviews with twenty nurses she was able to capture the rich views of experienced nurses. Specifically, the author discussed how nurses commit to colleagues, the employing institution, community, profession, and to self.

Rinaldi Carpenter (1989) found that nurses experience, importantly, commitment to each other. Nurses are motivated by small accomplishments which benefit others, not themselves. Their nature is to be self-sacrificing for the good of someone else. Since commitment needs to be nurtured, this nurturance must come not only from patients but from co-workers.

Commitment to the place nurses are employed is also evident. A sense of loyalty is manifested by how responsible nurses are in maintaining a professional demeanor both in appearance and in actions.

Nurses also experience a commitment to the health care needs of the community. The author noted that this experience of commitment is related to a recognition of the health care requirements of the community in which the nurse lives, and acceptance of responsibility in meeting those health care needs. This may require volunteer service on the part of the nurse in terms of public education and health screening, as well as a knowledge of available resources within the community. According to one of the subjects in Rinaldi Carpenter's study:

Helping the public, that's commitment too. Giving inservices . . . that's commitment. It's not just bedside nursing that you are committed to. It's the community, and teaching the public, teaching CPR, helping. That's commitment, helping people to understand. . . . That's commitment to the public.

Commitment is also experienced and manifested through participation in professional activities and in the professionalization of nursing. This commitment involves higher education, membership in professional organizations, and concern for the future of nursing. Commitment to the profession may also be perceived as having certain obstacles related to nursing as a female dominated profession. One such obstacle may be the need to strike a balance between professional commitments and home and family responsibilities. There is a perceived need to be committed to the nursing profession, and to unity within the profession, but nurses often find themselves pulled in many different directions.

Nurses experience a commitment to self. Although there is an innate, integral component of the nurse's personality which thrives on helping others and is fed by this experience, nurses often see a great deal of sadness, work without sufficient qualified help, and must deal day in and day out with the fact that they cannot do everything they want for their patients, students, or staff. At the same time nurses are dealing with the fact that the work also effects them as people. Lack of institutional support, inconvenient hours, working on advanced degrees and poor salary all wear on the emotional backbone of the nurse. Nurses in doctoral programs, in addition to experiencing work demands of a clinical nature, have strong fears and concerns about failing because they are overcommitted in many ways:

I am one third of the way into my PhD program—due soon for my candidacy. There is constant fear and talk among peers of not being able to "make it"—much of this is scare tactics. Nursing needs to help and support students—not scare, but mentor and assist.

I am originally a diploma graduate, graduating after completing a 2½-year program in 1971. My BSN (1975) was 138 credits—a 4 year curriculum taught in 4 calendar years. My MN (1978) was 52 credits (I went 2 years part time and 1 year full time). I originally began a PhD program in education and then switched to a PhD program in nursing. Due to a move, I started my third doctoral program, the current one, and have completed 10 credits thus far. I have a total of 208 college credits. In any other discipline, I would be a PhD plus! See if you can't end that craziness in nursing education!

The process of doctoral education is highly political and fraught with instances of inconsistency. I have been demoralized and reduced to tears by a few faculty members. Extremely stressful and somewhat inflexible.

Nursing at my doctoral program is struggling still to be thought of as an academic profession. The way they are managing this is to require more credits, more classes, and more work per class to complete the program than other disciplines. Obviously, I still find this worthwhile but I look forward to the day when we can relax a bit.

Nurses are committed to their professional roles and also to their personal roles. Nurses are primarily female. The social expectation has been for centuries that women will assume the nurturing role in society. Society is perceived to place value on things with dollar signs. The social reward for mothering or nurturing is perceived to be negligible (it is just expected).

Perhaps that is why many nurses seek the doctoral degree. They aspire to go beyond the nurturing role expected of them by society. They are committed to many things, but the commitment to self provides an inner drive to excel in the profession, learn all they can about the profession, and become scientists with a vision that practice can change or improve because of their commitment.

Doctoral education for nurses within the discipline of nursing is extremely important. I feel that nursing as a discipline is at a point developmentally where socialization of its own, rather than other disciplines such as education, sociology, etc. is critical. I feel that the purpose of doctoral education is primarily to train researchers; nurses who can further nursing knowledge.

As a first year doctoral student I have appreciated the emphasis on my worth as a scholar. The admission process was so rigorous that it is expected and accepted that we will succeed at doctoral studies. This has been a wonderful change from the extreme competition at baccalaureate and master's levels of preparation. I feel as if the university has been extremely attentive to our personal and professional needs. I am so pleased that I have made the commitment to this program. I feel as if I will be well prepared to deal with research and/or education careers on completion.

SUMMARY

Commitment prepares doctoral students to jump the many hurdles that will be expected of them when they begin their degree. The personal dedication, emotional investment and physical demands are consuming. Balancing family, school, and work becomes a norm. The commitments, in the words of Levenstein (1986) are complicated and numerous. The demands on one's human energy are complex. But in doctoral education, the rewards are plentiful—opened doors to career advancement, personal and professional growth and extreme satisfaction in achieving a life goal.

References

Clemence, M. (1966). Existentialism: a philosophy of commitment. *American Journal of Nursing, 3,* 500–505.

Gibran, K. (1951). *The prophet.* New York: Alfred A. Knopf.

Haughey, J. C. (1975). *Should anyone say forever?* New York: Doubleday and Company.

Levenstein, A. (1986). A contract of commitment. *Nursing Management, 17*(2), 75–76.

Merton, R. K. (1974). *The idea of social structure.* New York: Harcourt Brace.

Quinn, C. A., & Smith, M. D. (1987). *The professional commitment: Issues and ethics in nursing.* Philadelphia: W. B. Saunders.

Rinaldi Carpenter, D. M. (1989). *The lived experience of commitment to nursing: As perceived by nurses in a specific nursing environment* (unpublished doctoral dissertation).

Tourtillott, E. A. (1981). *Commitment—A lost characteristic?* New York: National League for Nursing Press, Pub. No. 23–1895.

van Manen, M. (1984). Practicing phenomenological writing. *Phenomenology and Pedagogy, 2,* 36–69.

CHAPTER EIGHT

On Jumping Hurdles

INTRODUCTION

IT BEGAN WITH a letter of acceptance following a rigorous application process. It didn't matter if you were employed full time, the head of a household, or a mother of three who would commute three hours after a tiring clinical day. An immediate love affair began with "the possibility" of achieving a lifetime goal—the doctorate in nursing. Somehow it would work out, the hurdles would be cleared, the hoops jumped—the ultimate in juggling acts accomplished. What was once an "idea" had become a reality.

Dealing with the logistics of attendance became a priority. You may never have been in Manhattan before or have driven to a big city, but now, somehow, you would—three times a week, and, after work. You will set short term goals as you ride along the interstate—"at the halfway mark I'll eat a candy bar, save the chicken sandwich for the wait at the bridge . . . M & M's are for the return trip—at 10 P.M. . . . I hope I can stay awake tonight! I really hope I never get a flat tire. Watch the deer alongside the road!"

A subway was once a foreign concept, but will soon become a best friend. You never dreamed you would know the parking lot attendants on a first name basis and exchange pleasantries for saving you a spot at 5 P.M. But that would soon happen.

The demands of work continue as you drive along. The staff meeting that needed better direction, the proposal to the Dean for more funding, or, the critically ill patients you would care for the next day. With your work day still on your mind you drive to class to learn how leaders in the nursing profession pursue their dreams.

Family concerns never leave you. The baby is sick but you are needed to present in a nursing theory debate. You are an integral part of class and must be there. So you sniffle (maybe cry) along the way to school, hoping the sitter will watch your little one and offer a hug or two or three until you return.

But is your mind totally there? Are you fully present in the classroom once you arrive? Although all the juggling has occurred and you are finally with your colleagues, you sit back and become absorbed in the issues of the profession, the research that impacts practice, and perhaps a stimulating presentation by a colleague on a cutting edge curriculum. You decide it is worth it.

The truth is, very few students can "just" go to school. Most have numerous commitments—family, work, research to name a few. So part-time study, which often includes a long commute to attend the doctoral program is a reality of achieving this degree.

The focus of this chapter is a discussion of the reality of doctoral education from the lived experience of students. Both qualitative and quantitative data are presented. Views on managing life commitments, maximizing the student experience, and issues such as access and finding the right match of program type are detailed.

Students have been extremely generous in sharing sincere commentary on the rigors of "doing it all." Going to school, nurturing a full-time career, sacrificing financially and socially, doing without sleep, being a wife, mother, or caregiver. Quite seriously, we have concern for those who wrote about their isolation, illness, lack of physical and emotional support. The challenge was painful and for some unbearable (they may never complete the degree). At times, the lack of access to the doctorate and inflexible nature of program planning was alarming. Many have looked back and said two words, never again.

All is not that dismal, however. The goal is so worth achieving, the rewards so satisfying that pride wins over pain. The magnificent learning and growth that occur as a leader and professional nurse are hard to measure. The student narratives that follow express the experiences of doctoral students in their own voices. Perhaps their message can offer comfort to those who seek this goal (plan to enroll) and to those seeking (enrolled). The anecdotes fall into four aspects; juggling it all, access, health and finances.

JUGGLE, JUGGLE—IN TOO DEEP?

Many students were not isolated in their need to juggle an extremely tiring, stressful, busy life. If they knew they were not alone in their pursuit however, they could support one another more effectively. A great need exists in doctoral programs to help individuals succeed, yet, make their lives less stressful.

I am in my second year of study in the doctoral program and am a part-time student. I also have a full-time job in research and work part-time as a nurse practitioner for a suburban health department (I've been there 17 years!). I find it difficult to balance all of this and still have a "personal life." I would love to be a full-time student and I am extremely excited about my course, yet I thoroughly enjoy my clinical work and feel I don't want to give that up either! The ideal of practice without research or research without practice, does not "fit" for me. Perhaps this struggle for me will become clearer as I progress in my studies—but right now I find myself trying to do everything!

I am on the faculty of one nursing program teaching at the undergraduate level and am a doctoral student at another (competing?) nursing program. The doctoral program does allow part-time students but does require two semesters of full-time study to establish residency. There is a double message; students are recruited to be in the program on a part-time basis, but once in, there is tremendous pressure to be available on campus for collegial relationships and projects with faculty. I have research mentors and a collegial network at my employing program and feel some tension between the expectation of the doctoral faculty and what my time will allow. I have a husband, children, and church activities that also require my energy and time. I pray a lot, juggle, and keep a list of all I need to do. The fatigue factor is tremendous. I do feel that despite the time constraints, I am receiving an excellent education and will grow as a nurse scientist.

The doctoral program that I am involved in is geared toward full-time students who either quit their jobs or are on leave and live on campus. I must work full-time and go to school part-time. I also commute two hours one-way to get to school. It is very difficult being a part-time student in a full-time student world. Courses are offered once a year or every other year. Student's PhD organization meets during the day. All guest speakers are during the day. Faculty office hours are once or twice a week and rarely on the day you are on campus. There is simply no support for those of us who commute and go to school part-time. It is greatly needed!

I do believe that the expectations of faculty that a doctoral student publish, teach and gain research experience (outside one's own dissertation/course work) while in the program, are difficult to meet because of real-life needs, such as family commitments and financial concerns. Compared to doctoral (PhD) students in other parts of the university, my peers and I are older and have more family commitments. We typically have practiced and taught for a number of years before entering doctoral study. Yet, the program seems geared to younger graduate students going straight through from the baccalaureate level. A greater acknowledgment of the diversity of student needs and strategies to accommodate these could maximize our performances in the program.

I think age is an issue to assess. Not that I have any regrets at all but if I had to do it over again, I'd do it around age 30–34 rather than 40.

As a part-time student, full-time worker (nursing administration), the "peer" component is less accessible and less important to me. Doctoral programs should be more directed to the needs and goals of part-time students who are advanced in their careers. "Immersion" is often not an option. I wanted doctoral preparation to be able to study and evaluate health care delivery processes and outcomes. I am getting very good preparation for that in my program.

I am a working student who cannot sacrifice family commitments/ mortgage for full-time study. I am, therefore, not on campus a great deal. Tradeoffs have included my lesser exposure to fellow doctoral students/informal support and education.

You should know that I have just started this quarter in a part-time capacity. I have two small children ages 3 and 5, and am working part-time in an innovative off-campus education program. My answers are based on limited impressions thus far with this program. One concern I have is the lack of support part-time students receive. If the "average" doctoral student is 38-years-old with 2.5 children and a complex life, then surely I am not the only one who finds it untenable to sever current professional and employment relations to pursue my studies full-time. The lack of financial support for part-time study is notable. I have a wonderful role model and faculty advisor and I hope this will develop into a mentor relationship.

I honestly don't have time to give this thoughtful consideration. I'm working full time, writing part time, and taking classes part time. I believe full-time study is an essential part of doctoral education, but it is really difficult to pull it off for the nontraditional student. A little flexibility (and a lot of funding) would be nice.

Most doctoral nursing students either have family responsibilities, work responsibilities or both. I am amazed by my peers who have both and carry a full course load. Of course, this is due to their maturity and to the nature of nurses to return to school after having spent a significant amount of time in the work force. I have mixed feelings about returning to school full time and working full time; I know the reality is that most of us cannot afford to quit our jobs for financial reasons, but I have always believed that if one chooses to return to school then school should take priority over work. Nursing education has not yet figured out how to deal with students who "do it all."

The biggest issue for me is how to balance full-time clinical responsibilities with teaching responsibilities and full-time student's responsibilities—there is no time left for me, and there is very little time to think and network informally. This should change dramatically when I'm done with course work, but for now I feel like I'm in too deep.

In summary, many nurses are just not willing to give up their clinical practice to singularly perform research or teach. They are not willing to give up the tenure of a secure job. They see a continued value and need in the profession to update clinical learning and the environments of patient care. They are mothers and fathers, wives and husbands who must work and cannot afford to be full-time students. They are responsible for both professional and personal commitments. Are they wrong in feeling they must balance these commitments? Should they end their careers to attend school full time? For many, doctoral education simply could not occur if not for part-time studies. As a profession it is very obvious from the accounts of students that we can no longer expect part-time students to adjust in a "full-time student world."

MAXIMIZING PERFORMANCE

So then, what will enable students in doctoral programs to succeed? First and foremost students deserve candid advice about the mission and philosophy of the program and if the program "fits" goals they have set forth. For example, if students have a clinical focus and want to pursue a doctoral program with a clinical science focus what program would be best? Most would say well of course, the DNS prepares the student for a clinical role. But, have differences between degree types been empirically measured? One student offered this anecdote:

> PhD programs need to be definitive and unwavering (unequivocally) in this regard (and must include mission statements that are not misleading to individuals). The majority of us are older, have families/ jobs/careers, and don't have time to spend a year or two of our lives finding out if the system we chose (or which chose us) is compatible with where we want to go in the future. I also believe that doctoral program educators need to be more candid about length of time in study and how much preparation a prospective PhD student needs before entering a program, especially if that individual has been out of school for a while.

FIT: WHAT PROGRAM BEST SUITS YOUR NEEDS?

In order to maximize student learning on the doctoral level, differences in program focus should be explained to students. In our national study on differences in students' perceptions reported in Chapter 2, we found differences by program type.

The authors conducted T-tests on two means from independent scales used. (Whether a pooled variance estimate was used depended on the results of the F-test for the equality of two variances.) The T-test was used to compare differences in the mean responses on each of the 36 variables in the visual analog scales. The results of the T-tests give a view of student perceptions in two areas: academic rigor and quality indicators.

ACADEMIC RIGOR

Measurement and Evaluation

In this component of the study, education was felt to be rigorous, particularly in measurement and statistics courses by all students. There was no significant difference between groups on this variable. Statistics courses were not taught by nursing faculty in most programs. Significant differences, however, were noted between the three groups of doctoral students on this variable. PhD ($p = .001$) and DNS ($p = .000$) nursing faculty taught statistics courses significantly more than EdD nursing faculty according to perceptions of students enrolled in these programs. When comparing PhD and DNS faculty, it was interesting to note that DNS nursing faculty were reported by DNS students to teach statistics more often than PhD faculty ($p = .034$).

Grade Point Average

Students generally perceived the grade point average (GPA) as being an easily managed component of doctoral education. EdD students agreed significantly more than PhD (p = .000) and DNS (p = .000) students that GPA was manageable. See Table 8.1.

Table 8.1 Academic Rigor									
Variable	PhD	DNS	Sig	EdD	DNS	Sig	EdD	PHd	Sig
Statistics Courses Were Rigorous	30	32	ns	20	32	ns	20	30	ns
GPA Manageable	35	36	ns	14	36	.000	14	35	.000
Statistics Taught by Nursing Faculty	80	66	ns	107	66	.000	107	80	.001

QUALITY INDICATORS

Teaching Excellence

Maintaining the quality of doctoral programs is an ongoing challenge as programs proliferate rapidly. Faculty excellence, teaching in doctoral programs, and the quality of education the students receive are widely discussed in the literature (Bremner, Crutchfield, Kosnowski, Perkins & Williams, 1990; Brodie, 1986; Casarett, 1989). Students in this study reported great satisfaction with the quality of their programs and the faculty. Respondents noted that faculty were actively engaged in research and frequently published in professional nursing journals.

Faculty Research

There were no significant differences between groups in response to active engagement in research. Significant differences, however, were reported in faculty publishing activities. PhD program faculty published in professional nursing journals significantly more than DNS faculty (p = .044). There was no significant difference between EdD and PhD faculty or EdD and DNS faculty on this variable.

Students learned "a great deal" from faculty in formal classroom settings. Participants also reported that strong mentorships existed in their programs, with EdD and PhD students agreeing more often than DNS students. The difference, however, was not significant.

Dissertation Support

All doctoral students generally agreed that dissertation support by nurse faculty was readily available. A significant difference was found, however, between PhD and DNS students, with PhD students reporting more dissertation support than their DNS colleagues (p = .050). EdD students also received significantly more support by nurse faculty on dissertations than DNS students surveyed (p = .027).

Students noted an adequate "series" of dissertation courses that prepared them for the dissertation project. There was no significant difference between PhD and DNS students on this variable. EdD students, however, differed considerably from PhD and DNS students, reporting significantly more dissertation preparation courses for dissertation projects than PhD (p = .000) and DNS (p = .000) students. See Table 8.2. There is little empirical evidence in the nursing literature that compares program types at the doctoral level in nursing. This lack of information leaves potential students inadequately informed. That is why our study is relevant. Similarities in program type have been reported (Snyder-Halpern, 1986; Ziemer, Brown, Fitzpatrick, Manfredi, O'Leary, & Valiga, 1992), however, significant differences have not been reported. We believe that our study demonstrates that differences exist. These differences should be noted and utilized by students seeking to understand subtle differences in program types.

In addition to doctoral students maximizing their performance by

Table 8.2		Quality Indicators							
	PhD	DNS	Sig	EdD	DNS	Sig	EdD	PhD	Sig
Faculty Research	20	27	ns	23	27	ns	23	20	ns
Faculty Publish	16	24	.044	21	24	ns	21	16	ns
Learn Faculty	24	31	ns	20	31	ns	20	24	ns
Dissertation Support	27	33	ns	19	33	.027	19	27	ns
Adequate Dissertation Courses	38	41	ns	15	41	.000	15	38	.000
Strong Mentorship Available	33	42	ns	30	42	ns	30	33	ns

finding the program that will enable their goals, faculty in these programs need to counsel and communicate with students regarding the curriculum and courses that will support their studies. Time frames must be explained realistically for program completion (doctoral faculty do know "ball park" time frames). Support available to students in the dissertation process must be clear. For example, are there courses that lead one to developing a dissertation proposal? Funding for education and research assistantships needs to be detailed. Finally, access to courses, faculty, and for example, equipment such as modems and other technology should be outlined. How many faculty have office hours in the night or are available on the weekends? Can one communicate with faculty via E-mail?

Access

Easy access would complement performance in doctoral education. Once students select a program that best fits their career goals, the question then becomes, is it accessible? Summer, night classes, one day programs, provision of reading materials in the classroom, are high on the list of means to facilitate learning in a doctoral program. A range of other possibilities needs serious consideration, such as teleconferencing, use of the Internet, and external site offerings. Doctoral students should question access to courses and support services. The need for innovative measures that facilitate student success as they juggle multiple responsibilities is vital. The following are student responses to program access:

> Doctoral education in nursing is not easily accessible, particularly for married individuals whose spouses and families cannot relocate to large university settings. Furthermore, even if more programs opened, there are not yet sufficient numbers of doctorally-prepared nurses to serve as faculty in them.

> Programs throughout the country do not generally work to meet the special needs of the doctoral student. Summers-only programs are scarce. Night classes are rare. Many schools will accept only full-time students, which is unrealistic for facilities requiring double incomes to pay mortgages etc. The closest school offering a doctoral degree for me is 2½ hours from my home. Fortunately, faculty are understanding and supportive. However, teleconferences and external site options would be extremely helpful and stress-reducing.

> The summers-only program was deleted after I started my doctoral program.

> Generally the positions of full-time student and full-time employee have been mutually exclusive. This mindset should be changed! The synergistic roles of employee-student should be encouraged, not discouraged.

> I continue to work full time while working toward my doctorate. Balancing work and school is difficult but manageable. Currently I attend full time, but during the two prior years I attended part time.

Offering part-time studies allows students to meet their educational as well as career growth needs. Income is important and essential and I would encourage more programs to consider options for part time.

Pertinent issues related to my education and to the doctoral program include a program which prepares one to be competent at the doctoral level upon completion of the program. This issue encompasses qualified faculty, curriculum and flexibility in program to meet student needs. Some specific areas include evening classes, provision of faculty assistance other than Monday through Friday business hours and well-staffed labs.

We must enhance accessibility to enable students to complete their doctoral education. One contemporary concept is the use of distance education to improve access, not only on the doctoral level but at the master's and BSN levels of nursing education, as well. Distance education programs are innovative competency-based methods that take into consideration the prior abilities and self-directedness of the student. For doctoral students, distance learning would provide access to, as well as, enhancement of adult learning objectives. Lewis and Farrell (1995) wrote in reference to distance education:

The underlying philosophy of this strategy includes the belief that when students have access to a program of planned instruction where the course materials are systematically designed and provide direction to additional resources, students can proceed in a self directed manner and be successful in meeting the specified outcomes for each course. The role of the teacher is that of facilitator and collaborator of the learning process rather than giver of information. These programs typically are described as correspondence, open learning/open university, semi-present, independent study/assessment, and, more recently, the electronic classroom. A common element in all these approaches to distance education is innovation in delivery of instruction and in teaching-learning methodologies, and little or no classroom time (p. 185).

The models of distance education are endless. For example, the California State University system, funded by W. K. Kellogg Foundations, created a distance education model for nurses in California. The Denver-based Mind Extension University (of Jones Intercable, Inc.,) offers courses via telecommunications and allows students the ability to register, pay for courses, order materials and access faculty and colleague voice mail. These examples of innovation could ultimately be the answer to access problems in doctoral education. The criteria fits well in that doctoral students are adult learners and self-motivated to complete objectives designed by the doctoral faculty (Johnston & Lewis, 1995).

But, let's simplify things a bit and talk about the outrageous! Access also refers to attention to the basics . . . day care, lodging, clinical site access (the observation of extant theory in practice, for example), creative funding and summer camp options. These "basics" apply to most students. Suppose your children could be taken care of while you study or go to the library? Is it outrageous to develop a modified child care program one day per week or on two evenings? How wonderful this would be for the children to meet other children from different states, and maybe different countries. How easy for the mom to know her children are being cared for in the very next building rather than 200 miles away.

Commuting students would also be comforted to know they could stay in a nearby hotel or dorm in case of inclement weather. Some programs may indeed arrange this, but do students know about this piece of security?

Summer learning, particularly for nursing faculty in the form of a camp or extended site would be well attended. An off-campus site for two weeks, where reading materials are provided, would be a welcome strategy for many who cannot afford to set aside one or two days a week throughout the school year.

Innovative access may be very energizing—albeit outrageous, but why not? Are doctoral nursing faculty so traditional and conventional that innovation is a dream? It is clear from the voices of the students that without creative access, many bright, gifted nurses will never experience advanced education on the doctoral level.

PERSONAL CRISES AND DOCTORAL EDUCATION

Good health, that is, physical and emotional health, is yet another hurdle among those in doctoral education. Students have written about personal crisis such as divorce, illness, and tremendous financial strain. One's personal life suffers. Family events change. Time is a critical factor. Although we haven't any statistics, we all know of colleagues who became divorced during pursuit of the doctorate. Relationships that were not on solid ground became increasingly jeopardized. Doctoral education is demanding and rigorous, frequently straining one's physical and emotional health. Often, the little time you have is divided among children, work, aging parents, and loved ones.

Much support and understanding are needed for everyone involved. Students must be particularly aware of the commitment and dedication required in their pursuit of the doctorate. Family and support systems must openly communicate to survive the demands of late nights at the computer, writing, or studying:

> I would like to suggest a study that would ask doctoral students in nursing about their physical health since entering their doctoral program. My program admits three to six doctoral students per year. Out of the six persons admitted in my class, one has died of a brain tumor, one developed a serious asthmatic condition, and two others have developed stress related symptoms. I know of at least two persons per class in the last five classes who have developed serious physical illnesses (heart palpitations, ulcerative colitis and anorexia). This tells the real story!

> This is the hardest thing I have every done in my life, but it has also been the best growth experience of my life. I find knowledge to be empowering, and I am overwhelmed when I think about all the new knowledge I have assimilated over the last few years. It also makes you see how little you know—quite humbling! I have been fortu-

nate, although school has been very difficult for me and I have struggled, I have done better than I expected. One of the things that was the most difficult for me was that I began to question my ability to do the course work, and in the process lost my self-confidence. It has taken me a year to "pull myself back together" again.

I do believe that doctoral study does take an emotional toll. I feel that instead of increasing my self-confidence it has actually decreased my self-confidence.

Emotional and physical changes in the health of students are a reality. Are those educating doctoral students aware of the health alterations among class members? Are they too busy to take an interest? Are students more concerned about succeeding than their health? The tremendous dedication by doctoral students is astounding . . . but is it healthful?

Another layer of concern is financing doctoral education. One husband of a recent graduate commented that it was like "putting a child through college but on a more grandiose scale." Financial burden is relevant and having to take leave from a job to complete a doctoral program is quite costly. Funding is limited and in some programs "nonexistent." In the schools that have grant funding, students commented on how helpful this assistance truly was . . . but most paid from their own pocket.

As a single parent of two, I have found the lack of financial assistance very difficult. When one is admitted to any PhD program, the highest level you can be employed at is a TA/RA for $10–$11 dollars/hr. I couldn't support my family on that (and no health/dental benefits were available for dependents). Grants are basically for equipment and limit your employment to 25 percent. Once again, not practical for single parents. Perhaps I'm extra tired tonight, but I have found it difficult to balance full-time work (plus the five consulting and part time jobs), parenthood (but the kids are doing great!!) and school. I managed to get course work done; the next year, completed the three written prelims; and the next year, passed orals but I'm having a rough time getting my proposal pulled together. It is difficult to get blocks of time to work on it and my research is clinically based, so it will take a while to collect data. . . . therefore, the majority of nurses continue to be female. Many females are single parents needing food and shelter for their families. Current funding is not adequate to meet the basic needs of these families and so the student/parent is on constant overload. I wonder how many bright nurses look at the "costs" of doctoral education, shake their heads, and with a sigh, say "I just can't do it!"

Because my income is high enough with six jobs, I don't need much money, according to accountant, etc. I've tried to explain that although my tax statement does reflect an adequate income it would be nice to just work one job or maybe even .8 and get done with school. That logic doesn't seem to cut it . . . sigh!

Money has been a difficult problem for me during my studies since I am from out-of-state and am the head of the household. The Dean of the program is a sensitive, supportive lady. She sets a supportive tone for the program.

Funding to support doctoral students is scarce and competitive. It will be a long time before doctoral education in nursing will be widespread.

Grant funding at my school tremendously eases the financial burden for me. I'd have to work while going to school if funding wasn't available. The dual roles (job and school) would make it difficult to devote attention to both in any pattern of fairness.

A huge issue that needs to be addressed is the lack of funding to support education of doctorally prepared RNs. There needs to be better federal and state support of nurses since the shortage of doctorally prepared nurses is so critical.

Doctoral education is a personal and heavy financial problem involving living away from home, resigning faculty positions, and taking out loans.

SUMMARY

The numerous burdens of the doctoral education process must be addressed. In this chapter, the rigors of trying to "do it all" were discussed: nurturing a career, sacrificing personally and financially, finding a program that is best, accessing doctoral education, and noting personal crises that may occur. Students seeking doctoral education should have an awareness of the multiple demands in order to prepare themselves and their families. Being aware and being informed will help students succeed in clearing the hurdles.

References

Bremner, M., Crutchfield, A., Kosnowski, M., Perkins, J., & Williams, G. (1990). Doctoral preparation of nursing faculty. *Nurse Educator, 15,* 12–15.

Brodie, B. (1986). Impact of doctoral programs on nursing education. *Journal of Professional Nursing, 2,* 350–357.

Casarett, A. (1989). Components needed to support graduate education. *Journal of Professional Nursing, 5,* 256–260.

Johnston, M. K., & Lewis, J. (1995). Reaching RNs through the electronic classroom. *Nursing and Health Care: Perspectives on Community, 16*(4), 237–238.

Lewis, J. M., & Farrell, M. (1995). Distance Education: A strategy for leadership development. *Nursing and Health Care: Perspectives on Community 16*(4), 184–187.

Hudacek, S., & Carpenter, D. R. (1994). Doctoral education in nursing. *Review of Research in Nursing Education, VI.* New York: National League for Nursing Press, Pub. No. 19-2544.

Hudacek, S., & Carpenter, D. (1995). The Chameleon Connection. Manuscript submitted for publication.

Snyder-Halpern, R. (1986). Nursing doctorates: Is there a difference? *Nursing Outlook, 34,* 284–286.

Ziemer, M., Brown, J., Fitzpatrick, M. L., Manfredi, C., O'Leary, J., & Valiga, T. (1992). Doctoral programs in nursing: Philosophy, curricula, and program requirements. *Journal of Professional Nursing, 8*(1), 56–62.

CHAPTER NINE

On Growing

Grow, Stretch . . . You Can Do It!

Student Comment

INTRODUCTION

THE PRECEDING CHAPTERS demonstrate that doctoral education is a multifaceted process which contributes to the individual's personal and professional growth. The many facets of doctoral education impact the individual in both positive and negative ways and may contribute to significant life changes. This chapter summarizes the multiple aspects of doctoral education and highlights key areas of personal and professional growth.

PERSONAL GROWTH

The process of doctoral education affects the individual from the moment the application process begins, to the time when the first foot is set on campus. Almost before one knows what one is getting into personal sacrifices are made. It matters very little whether you are talking about an individual with a husband and children, or a single career person, sacrifice is made in one's personal life in an attempt to complete this process. Personal time, family time, work time, and relaxation all are pushed aside as an attempt is made to complete the grueling process. Van Dongen (1988), in a qualitative study on the life experience of the first year doctoral students noted:

> Changes and losses in social and recreational activities were also experienced by all subjects. There was a definite reduction in the amount of time spent socializing with others. Students described carefully "screening" potential social events in terms of whether they could be accommodated in their schedule. Time devoted to community activities, professional organizations, and personal hobbies was also sharply curtailed or discontinued entirely. One student stated, "My life used to be colorful and diverse like a calico quilt, but not as a doctoral student, it's like a gray army blanket . . . still warm, but definitely less colorful." All students interviewed also spontaneously reported often experiencing feelings of guilt when they spent time doing "nondoctoral" activities (p. 22).

Doctoral study has also been noted to be a source of marital conflict among married students. The rate of divorce among doctoral students and individuals with doctorates has been found to be higher than in the general population (Fischer, 1981). Con (1983) explored burnout among married and single students and found higher levels of emotional exhaustion among married students.

Budgeting one's time becomes very important early in the doctoral education process. Leisure time, time to read the newspaper or watch your local news is now filled with other responsibilities. An hour in between teaching a class or taking a class can be used to critique a paper or review needed references for a project in the library. Getting up an hour or two earlier, and going to sleep an hour or two later changes the personal life of the doctoral student dramatically but is needed time to finish classroom or work-related responsibilities. Very few doctoral students are simply "doing the doctorate." Most are juggling many responsibilities and personal sacrifices are made in order to succeed. Heins, Fahey, and Leiden (1984) noted that the prime sources of stress for medical, law and graduate students were inadequate time and economic pressures. Urbano (1986) described a developmental process experienced by doctoral students that involved an initial adjustment period marked by anxiety and dissonance. Later in the process the student is required to become an increasingly independent learner, disciplining oneself to conduct the dissertation research, and finally completing the degree.

Learning from other students and from one's mentor about the "need to knows" and the "nice to knows" is critical. This type of inside track knowledge helps the student cope with the many projects and responsibilities that have been assumed and contributes to the learning of how to budget one's time efficiently. Completing the doctoral education process is not only about being intellectually capable but it is also about being disciplined and organized in one's work. This discipline must be learned early on if one is to finish the dissertation and not end up All But Degree (ABD). Course work supplies some built-in structure for the student, but completing the dissertation will require that the student be self-directed, organized and independent in completion of the work. Although many students will arrive in the doctoral programs with these personal attributes, many will need to develop these skills throughout their course work. As Van Dongen (1988) noted:

> Students typically worked a nonstop 17-hour day that included diverse family and student responsibilities. Subjects described the need to "make every minute count" and routinely strived to accomplish several activities simultaneously, i.e., cook dinner, supervise the children, do laundry, and think about the next assignment due for class (p. 22).

Doctoral education seems like an arduous task that takes its toll on the individual's personal life. Most doctoral students do, however, find the personal sacrifices to be worthwhile in the ultimate achievement of the goal of completing the doctorate. The following narrative comments highlight aspects of personal growth as viewed by doctoral students.

Personal Growth

At this point, integrity and maturity are a prerequisite to academic success.

Self-confidence and self-esteem must add to and augment personal growth even for those who arrive confident and secure in their abilities.

Doctoral education really hasn't affected my overall self-confidence.

I feel that instead of increasing my self-confidence, it has actually decreased my self-confidence.

A very growth-producing experience.

I found doctoral education to be a rich and rewarding experience which changed my life.

The process of doctoral education in its goal of "reshaping" the individual, is destructive to self-esteem.

PROFESSIONAL GROWTH

Career mobility is often a motivational force for students enrolling in doctoral programs. Anyone in higher education knows that without the almighty doctorate, promotion and tenure are only a dream. If one is planning on entering or staying in academia for very long, achievement of the doctoral degree is a requirement. Promotion and tenure in the university system generally do not exist for those who are not doctorally prepared. Further, research requirements of faculty at most universities require that the individual be prepared at the doctoral level. Expanding and developing one's ability to conduct independent research is also an important aspect of the professional growth that occurs for the individual engaged in doctoral study. Doctoral students soon discover that, "in every class discussion and in every contribution that we made to the discussions following meetings, seminars, or guest lectures, we were being pressed, guided, and groomed to use the analytical skills of the scholar" (Johnson, Moorhead, & Daly, 1992, p. 280).

Professional growth at the doctoral level has as its central focus the development of scholarly points of view and the ability to conduct research. Further, one broadens and sharpens their perspectives about nursing in general. Most importantly, one makes a commitment to lifelong learning and develops a professional sense of the fact that there is no end to learning and the development of a scholar. Leddy and Pepper (1989) noted that as doctoral students a commitment is made to emulate the person of the scholar. This implies that we redefine our self-image to the point that we learn to feel and behave as scholars. This process occurs through mentoring, networking, and curricular course work. Doctoral students noted the following regarding professional growth:

PROFESSIONAL GROWTH

Preparation is directed toward excellence, but excellence rests ultimately with the researchers, their ethical sense and ability to pursue the goal of a doctorate.

I enjoy the opportunity to stretch and strengthen my abilities in a highly scholarly environment.

My ability to be a critical thinker, and increase my self confidence in terms of professional abilities was of utmost importance.

Self-confidence in doing specific research tasks has increased.

The first year of my PhD program decreased my self-confidence. Loss of clinical role where expertise was recognized was decreased.

Being doctorally prepared has reinforced why I love nursing.

Achieving my PhD represents a significant personal and professional goal for me.

I have grown both personally and professionally.

The doctorate did not help my confidence in nursing. It's the old adage: the more we know the more we realize we don't know.

Motivation and perseverance are difficult to quantify but are more important than GPA, GRE's or any other standard for prediction of outcome in doctoral education.

A person gets from a program exactly what he/she puts into it.

Life experiences can significantly contribute to how one approaches doctoral education.

The rigor of doctoral studies must be made even more difficult by the self-doubt that attends students and is only slightly mediated by the successful completion of candidacy.

SUMMARY

Doctoral education influences the lives of students in many different ways. All aspects of the process change the individual both personally and professionally. Mentoring, networking, curricular components and research methods all impact on the professional growth of the student. What the student gets out of a program has a great deal to do with what the student puts into the process, as well as the student's level of commitment to earning the doctorate. Whether positive or negative experiences occur all contribute to the student's personal growth. Utimately, the process of doctoral education should prepare leaders who are excited about the profession and the important contributions they are now prepared to make.

References

Con, E. H. (1983). Life style correlates of graduate student burnout. *Dissertation Abstract International, 44(B):* 1955.

Fischer, S. E. (1981). Quality of life, adjustment and stress among graduate students. *Dissertation Abstracts International, 44(B):* 3187.

Heins, M., Fahey, S., & Leiden, L. (1984). Perceived stress in medical, law, and graduate students. *Journal of Medical Education, 59,* 169–79.

Johnson, R. A., Moorhead, S. A., & Daly, J. M. (1992). Scholarship and socialization: Reflections on the first year of doctoral study. *Journal of Nursing Education, 31*(6), 280–282.

Leddy, S., & Pepper, J. M. (1989). *Conceptual bases of professional nursing.* Philadelphia: J. B. Lippincott.

Urbano, M. T. (1986). A developmental approach to doctoral education. *Journal of Nursing Education, 25,* 76–78.

Van Dongen, C. J. (1988). The life experience of the first-year doctoral student. *Nurse Educator, 13*(5), 19–24.

Appendix A
Doctoral Dissertations in Nursing from 1990–1994: A Selected Chronological Listing According to Topic

These titles were published over a period of five years by Sigma Theta Tau. They represent the trends in nursing research doctoral studies within that time frame. See Chapter 6 for analysis.

WOMEN'S ISSUES: 1990

1. The lived experience of fear in battered women.
2. The relationship between selected variables and the self-esteem of adolescent females.
3. Giving up: Shelter experiences of battered women.
4. A description of the maternal decision-making process regarding circumcision.
5. The process of bereavement for Mexican-American widows: A grounded theory.
6. Childbirth pain communicative behaviors among selected Thai women.
7. The impact of the hospital environment on early maternal mood state.
8. Effects of sustained nurse/mother contact on infant outcomes among low income African-American families.

9. Using self-efficacy to explain maternal confidence during toddlerhood.

10. Risk reduction in sexual behaviors of divorced and separated women.

11. An analysis of social networks as factors influencing social support among depressed women.

12. Control and satisfaction with the birth experience.

13. The experience of the perimenopause among Botswana women.

14. The health assessment of older women interview guide health sources component: A psychometric evaluation.

15. A study of parents' perceptions of the miscarriage experience.

16. The relationship between social support and postpartum depression.

17. Temperament and mother-child attachment.

18. Psychophysiological correlates of fatigue during childbirth.

19. Measurement of clinical decision-making by the nursing comps, the twelve point postpartal check microcomputer simulation.

20. The use of exercise to increase joint mobility in females 62 years of age and older.

21. The relationship of expertise to views of quality of nursing care for hospitalized prenatal women.

22. Cultural care, cultural health and grief phenomena related to older Greek Canadian widows within Leininger's Theory of Culture Care.

23. The experience of being homeless: A phenomenological study of homeless women.

24. Relationship of health benefits and self-efficacy to the practice of breast self-examination in adult women.

25. The influence of maternal attachment and the capacity for empathy on perception of social support among pregnant minority women.

26. Social support network structure and psychological function in adolescent mothers and delayers: A longitudinal study.

27. Reminiscences of elderly females.

28. Separation loss in searching birthmothers.

29. Gynecologic cancer as crisis: Predictors of adjustment.

30. Breast engorgement in breastfeeding mothers.

31. Effect of nurse-client transaction on female adolescents' contraceptive perceptions and adherence.

32. Caregiver burden and adaptation in middle-aged daughters of dependent, elderly parents: A test of Roy's Model.

33. Breast self-examination: A test of Decis' Theory of self-determination.

34. Factors that influenced the career decision of maternal-child nurses.

35. Coping and social support in a group of widows.

36. Cohesive experiences of young women in support groups: A phenomenological study.

37. Subjective experiences of leisure among older black women.

38. Indices of attachment in elderly women not mentally compromised residing in nursing homes.

39. Effect of movement group therapy on depression, morale, and self-esteem in aged women.

40. Women's dependence and independence during late antepartum through postpartum.

41. Perceived health status, perceived stress, and family satisfaction of wives of alcoholics and of non-alcoholics.

42. Experience of parenthood for adolescent mothers with toddlers.

43. Women's explanations for depression.

44. The knowledge of menopause: An analysis of scientific and everyday discourses.

45. Health status and psychological well-being in elderly women: The self-system as mediator.

46. Exploratory study of the sociocultural factors in depression among women in Southeast India.

WOMEN'S ISSUES: 1991

1. Differences in the frequency of use of breast cancer control methods in black and white women: An application of the Health Belief Model.

2. The process of recovering in women who have been depressed.

3. Health promoting behaviors of married and unmarried mothers.

4. Correlates of self-transcendence in women with advanced breast cancer.

5. Caregiving, approval, and family functioning in families with adolescent mothers.

6. Developmental aspects of pregnancy: Correlates of self-satisfaction.

7. Pain response in Mexican-American and white non-Hispanic women following a cholecystectomy.

8. Homeless womens' holistic and family planning needs: An exposition and test of the Nurse Practitioner Practice Model.

9. A woman for all seasons: A biography of Julia Catherine Stimson.

10. A descriptive study of biopsychosocial factors affecting adolescent female sexual activity in a multicultural population.

11. Role, status changes, and family planning use among Cambodian refugee women.

12. The mature gravida's orchestration of pregnancy from conceiving to birthing.

13. Validating women's experiences of living with chronic non-malignant pain.

14. Moral decision-making factors and caregiver burden in employed women caring for incapacitated parents.

15. Alteration in the body image of adolescent females braced as a treatment for adolescent idiopathic scoliosis.

16. An exploration of understandings of spirituality among women in Appalachia.

17. Coping strategies and women's development during the Age 30 Transition.

18. The postpartum experience: A study of maternal concerns, confidence, and support.

19. Testing a model of coping effectiveness in older women.

20. Effects of self-esteem, threat appraisal, and coping responses on the somatic components of illness: A test of a proposed causal model with professional women.

21. Mothers and adult daughters: Self-differentiation, attachment and mental state.

22. A study of maternal employment and family contexts: Influences on maternal health and mother-infant interaction.

23. The effect of discrete muscle activity on stress response.

24. Advocating for self: A grounded theory of women's process of fertility regulation.

25. A longitudinal study of cortical bone loss in white women.

26. Ill fate: Women's illness experiences in the pluralistic health care system of Taiwan.

27. Development of an instrument to measure satisfaction with patient care in the postpartum period.

28. The meaning of phenomena influencing adoption as an option for pregnant adolescents.

29. The relationship of depression and type of bereavement, mode of death, and time since death in three groups of adult females.

30. Women's experiences losing weight and gaining the lost weight back.

31. Age, social support, and the development of maternal behaviors in first-time teen and first-time non-teen mothers.

32. Self-coherence, coping, and mood in women following a hysterectomy.

33. The effects of aerobic exercise training on symptomatic females with mitral valve prolapse.

34. A comparison of grief responses and physical health changes in Caucasian and African-American women following a third trimester stillbirth.

35. Abused women's cognitive beliefs associated with readiness to terminate the relationship.

36. Stages of ego development: Relationships with personal autonomy and professional autonomy in female baccalaureate nursing students.

37. Development of self-concept during the three trimesters of pregnancy.

38. Patterns and processes of physical activity among black working women: An ethnographic study.

39. Perceived health status, spiritual well-being, and selected health practices among Mexican-American women.

40. Maternal-child home visiting: Elements of a public health nursing program.

41. Long distance Japanese marriages: Maintaining harmony during separation.

WOMEN'S ISSUES: 1992

1. Pregnancy in prison.

2. Cognitive response to symptoms in women with rheumatoid arthritis.

3. Homeless women's holistic and family planning needs: An exposition and test of the Nurse Practitioner Model.

4. Being pregnant and using drugs: A retrospective phenomenological inquiry.

5. Factors influencing a battered women's perception of controllability in violent relationships.

6. Home management of preterm labor: The negotiation of activity restriction.

7. Lesbian's experiences with alcohol problems: A critical ethnographic study of problematization, help-seeking, and recovery patterns.

8. A grounded theory study of conditions and processes of supportive interactions for single mothers.

9. Men who are caregivers of cognitively impaired wives: Becoming imbedded in the role.

10. Impact of the marital relationship and infant temperament on symptom distress in the postpartum period.

11. Impact of a woman's perception of labor and delivery, emotional stress, partner support, and sense of mastery on maternal depression symptoms reported at four weeks postpartum.

12. Health care experiences of a racially and economically diverse group of lesbians: A feminist narrative study.

13. Moving toward harmony: Types and meanings of cues that prompt health promoting decisions in women in the middle years.

14. A phenomenological study of women with AIDS who contracted HIV through heterosexual transmission.

15. The criminal prosecution of mothers of drug exposed neonates: A case study of a policy dilemma.

16. Being homeless: An ethnographic study of women's experiences in a shelter.

17. A prospective study documenting women's experiences combining breastfeeding and employment.

18. Perinatal depressive symptoms, quality of life, social support, and risk factors in Mexican-American women.
19. Self-presentation and minority women: Exploring psychosocial factors that influence health practices of African-American women.
20. Investigation intention to breastfeed: Applying the Triandis Model of Social Behavior.
21. Women's perceptions of tubal ligation.
22. Biological and psychological differences among first-episode and recurrently depressed women during depression and recovery.
23. Patterns of feminine and self-concept scores of pregnant women from the third trimester to six weeks postpartum.
24. Health promotion self-care actions of healthy, middle-aged women.
25. The relationship of power and feminism in female nurse executives in acute care hospitals.
26. The relationship between maternal depression, self-esteem, and mothers' perception of the temperament of their infants.
27. Induced elective abortion and perinatal grief.
28. The nature of the experience of women caregivers for aged parents: A social problem.
29. Life events stress, social support, and maternal-fetal attachment in incarcerated pregnant women and non-incarcerated pregnant women.
30. Correlates of depressive symptomatology in Korean-American women in New York.
31. Early intrapartal childbirth preparation, self-coherence, and physical and psychological outcomes of labor.
32. Emotional distress, coping behaviors and immunity in women undergoing breast biopsy.
33. The lived experience of Oregon Mexican-American women with diabetes and selected family members.

34. Recognition on maternal identity in pre-term and full-term mothers.

35. Filipino women's morale and mood: Their relationships with appraisal of and coping with the political instability in the Philippines.

36. Patterns of change in primipara's moods and functional status: An extension of Rubin's Nursing Model.

37. Health promotion behavior: The relationship with health conception, health perception, and self-esteem in obese women.

38. Attachments between mothers and their adopted children.

39. Protecting hearth and health: Hero women's sacred calling and secret burden.

40. Determining treatment for women with early breast cancer: Physician's perspectives.

WOMEN'S ISSUES: 1993

1. Multiple roles and health promotion lifestyles of women nurse educators.

2. Taking care: Taking care of self, taking care of others: Female chemically dependent nurses.

3. Patterns of appraisal, coping, emotions, and indices of recovery during the hysterectomy experience.

4. Relationships of selected physiological, psychosocial, and spiritual variables associated with survivorship in African-American women with breast cancer.

5. Seeking a healthy baby: Hispanic women's views of pregnancy and prenatal care.

6. Perceived psychological stress, perceived adequacy of social networks of first-time mothers 20–25 and 30–35 years of age.

7. Professional nurse and generic care of childbirthing women conceptualized within Leininger's Culture Care Theory and using Colaizzi's Phenomenological Method.

8. Menstrual self-care of collegiate athletes.

9. The relationship between self-efficacy, satisfaction with birth experience, postnatal stress response and childbirth education attendance in an obstetrical clinic population.

10. Relationship between feminine hygiene practices, body image, and self-esteem.

11. Thinking ability of women in nursing.

12. Wives' perceptions of situational experiences during critical care hospitalization: A phenomenological study.

13. Understanding decision making in the caregiving experience of mothers and daughters.

WOMEN'S ISSUES: 1994

1. Self-esteem, sense of mastery, and adequacy of pre-natal care.

2. An exploration of the physical and psychological responses of surgically-induced menopausal Saudi women using the Neuman System.

3. The effect of social support on women's perception of peri-menstrual changes.

4. Physiological and psychological distress: A descriptive study of nulliparous women who develop ketonuria during labor.

5. Factors that influence the diet and exercise behaviors and experiences of immigrant Mexican women.

6. Effects of employment and social support on first-time mothers age 30 and older the first year of motherhood.

7. Life as experienced by women in their 60's: A phenomenologic/Hermeneutic Study.

8. Women's experience of laboring in water.

9. Afro-American women's perspectives on motherhood.

10. The Urban Poor African-American woman's perceptions and experiences with prenatal care: A phenomenological study.

11. Relationship among prenatal maternal attachment, post-natal depressive symptoms and maternal role attainment.

12. Mammography: Predisposing, enabling, and need variables.

13. The post-hysterectomy experience of women: A cross-sectional study.

14. The effects of maternal psychosocial factors on parenting.

15. Women's self-efficacy for the prevention of sexual risk behavior.

16. Mothers' interpretations of their children's behavior during mother-child interaction.

17. An analysis of the experience of surviving and having children after breast cancer.

18. The effect of a 6KG weight load on functional capacity, body composition, and the lipid profile of middle-aged women.

19. Relationship among health state factors, foundational capabilities, and urinary incontinence self-care in women.

20. Basic conditioning factors and self-care agency of unmarried women at risk for sexually transmitted disease.

21. Women's experiences using terbutaline pump therapy for the management of preterm labor.

22. The meaning of being in preterm labor: A Hermeneutic Inquiry.

23. Health care encounters of women in abusive relationships: A process of protecting personal integrity.

24. An analysis of the costs and effects of three levels of maternity services in West Philadelphia.

25. The prevalence of and psychosocial factors associated with postpartum depression of mothers in Taiwan.

26. The meaning of launching a child: Women's mid-life as context for transition.

27. Body image dissatisfaction, sex-role identity, and self-esteem in mid-life women.

28. Women undergoing pelvic extenteration with vaginal reconstruction.

29. Interventions with employed mothers of infants: Effects on perceived stress, perceived social support, and parental competence.

30. Health beliefs, health focus of control, self-efficacy and self-examination behaviors among adult African-American women.

31. Midlife women's balanced health and ability to function through the process of self-care.

32. Personal meanings of control reported by women in their birth stories: A feminist perspective.

CARDIAC: 1990

1. The effects of two methods of dangling on heart rate and blood pressure in postoperative abdominal hysterectomy patients.

2. The influence of self-selected monotonous sounds on the night sleep patterns of post-operative open heart surgery patients.

3. Impact of stress and coping on adherence and health status in patients with hypertension.

4. Life after stroke: Survivor's bodily and practical knowledge of coping during recovery.

5. Physiologic and behavioral responses to acute myocardial ischemic pain in Mexican male patients.

6. The relationship between physiologic variables affected by open heart surgery and patient memory in the first post-op month.

7. Functional capacity: Coronary patients' participation in supervised versus unsupervised exercise training.

8. Coping with acute myocardial infarction.

9. Indicators of sympathetic nervous system overactivity in hypertensives.

10. The effects of sense of control, social support, and coping behavior on short-term adaptational outcomes for post-myocardial infarction clients.

11. Coronary and aortic vascular responsiveness to endothelin in the guinea pig.

12. Uncertainty and coping following coronary artery bypass surgery.

13. The relationships between adherence to cardiac rehabilitation, self-efficacy, anxiety, and activity tolerance.

14. Circulatory response following coronary artery bypass grafting.

15. Circadian rhythm of blood pressure in school-age children of normotensive and hyper-tensive parents.

CARDIAC: 1991

1. Social support and compliance after completion of a cardiac rehabilitation program.

2. Social support and cardiac invalidism following acute myocardial infarction.

3. Predictors of activity levels in patients with congestive heart failure.

4. Effects of time on lifestyle adjustments following a cardiac event as influenced by an outpatient cardiac rehabilitation program.

5. Self-efficacy and mood status in recovery from percutaneous transluminal coronary angioplasty.

6. Uncertainty and coping following coronary artery bypass surgery.

7. Stress, social support, psychological distress, and well-being in older women with chronic heart disease.

8. The relationship of the taxonomy conditions that necessitate nursing care in relations to outcomes in the cardiovascular surgical patient.

9. Temporal patterns of heart rate and rhythm, stroke volume, and cardiac output in critically ill adults in a cardiac surgical intensive care unit.

10. The relationship between causal attributions adjustment and coping in patients following a myocardial infarction.

11. Effects of preparation methods to enhance coping with cardiac catheterization among hospitalized school-aged Korean children.

12. The effect of nursing follow-up on self-care behaviors of post myocardial infarction patients.

13. Effect of length of counting interval and method of measurement on the accuracy of heart rate assessment in atrial fibrillation.

14. A community-based educational approach to enhance learning outcomes in black hypertension patients.

15. Children's cardiovascular health promotion attitude scale: An instrument development.

16. Recovery following sudden cardiac death during hospitalization.

CARDIAC: 1992

1. Life on hold: A theory of spouse response to the waiting period prior to heart transplantations.

2. Effects of a combined biofeedback relaxation intervention and oxygen consumption in patients with advanced heart failure.

3. Patterns of heart rate variability.

4. Psychosocial correlates of cardiac recovery.

5. Value of MCL1, MCL6, and selected ECG leads in the diagnosis of wide QRS complex tachycardia.

6. Quality of life in post-myocardial infarction women.

7. Cardiac patients' stress appraisals, emotions, and coping.

8. The lived experience of help-seeking in spouses of cardiac patients.

9. Cognitive appraisal of psychological stress, appraisal contexts, and life disruption in patients having percutaneous transluminal coronary angioplasty.

10. Coronary heart disease and cardiac arrest survival: sense of coherence as a predictor of quality of life.

11. Multi-dimensional scaling analysis of self-care actions for reintegrating holistic health after a myocardial infarction: Implications for nursing.

12. An exploratory descriptive study of physiological variables and the nursing diagnosis powerlessness in a population of intra-aortic balloon pumped patients.

13. The family experience following acute myocardial infarction.

CARDIAC: 1993

1. The effect of selected variables during the college experience on cardiovascular risk.

2. Left ventricular function in men during cognitive stress before and after coronary artery bypass grafts.

3. The experience of quality of life after coronary artery bypass surgery.

4. Recovery in the elderly after coronary artery bypass surgery.

5. Cardiovascular disease risk factors in adolescent male football athletes and other adolescent males.

6. Relationship among self care knowledge, self care resources, activity level and life satisfaction in persons three to six months after a myocardial infarction.

7. Exopolysaccharides of streptococcus mutants are virulence factors in dental caries and endocarditis.

CARDIAC: 1994

1. Relationship among subjective mental workload, experience, and education of cardiovascular critical care registered nurses.

2. The experiences of Taiwanese patients during recovery transition from cardiac surgery.

3. Factors related to long-term physical activity following coronary bypass graft surgery.

4. An investigation of a nursing system to support nutritional self-care in post myocardial infarction patients.

5. Patient-controlled access to visitation in the coronary care unit.

6. The relationships of self-motivation and perceived personal competence to engaging in a health-promoting lifestyle for men in cardiac rehabilitation programs.

7. Effects of a self-efficacy intervention on adherence to anti-hypertensive regimens.

8. Effect of an information intervention on recovery outcomes of patients and spouses following coronary artery bypass graft surgery.

9. Convalescence after cardiac surgery: A dyadic experience.

10. Factors predicting health behaviors in women with coronary heart disease and their family members.

11. Determinants of exercise behavior after myocardial infarction.

12. Developing a scale to measure responses of clients with actual or potential myocardial infarctions.

13. Study of intra-aortic balloon pumped patients.

14. Nursing intensity for acute myocardial infarction (DRG's 121 and 122) who were discharged.

THE ELDERLY: 1990

1. Structural-functional aspects of caring for elders in home environment.
2. Selected variables associated with falling in a male geriatric rehabilitation and long-term care setting.
3. The meaning of adult day care within the context of the caregiving relationship: Perspectives of older adults and their female caregivers.
4. Power, creativity, and reminiscence in the elderly.
5. Caregiver expectations of future learning by their older retarded dependents.
6. The use and acceptance of touch by elderly nursing home residents and their caregivers.
7. Interrelationships of religiosity, social resources, coping responses, health and well-being among older adults.
8. Feelings in relation to intrusions of territory and personal space of the nursing home resident.
9. Self-care practices and health status of individuals over the age of 55.
10. Communicating with residents with Alzheimer's Dementia: A study of nurse/resident interactive behavior.
11. Care and cure meanings, experiences and orientations of persons who are dying in hospital and hospice settings.
12. The phenomenon of care in high context culture: The old order Amish.
13. The relationship between stimulation programs and their frequency on depression in institutionalized geriatric clients.

14. An investigation of the relationship of hardiness and death attitudes to depression in older persons in skilled nursing facilities.

15. An investigation of the relationships of life satisfaction, purpose in life, and love in persons 65 years and older.

16. Interpersonal factors and nursing home resident health.

17. Rural/urban differences in health care needs of elderly discharged from hospital to home.

18. The relationship between loneliness, social support, and decline in cognitive function in hospitalized aged men and women.

19. The relationships among coping, hardiness, and outcomes of multiple chronic illnesses in the elderly.

20. Relationships between depression, self-esteem, and loneliness in elderly community residents.

21. Health promoting self-care behavior in the community older adult.

22. Spatial temporal experiences and self-assessed health in the older adult.

23. Appraisal, social distance, and the informal caregiver's multidimensional cost of caring for an elder family member.

24. Subjective perceptions of the demands of hospitalization and anxiety in bone marrow transplant patients.

25. Respite for kin caregivers of cognitively impaired elders.

ELDERLY: 1991

1. Functional status as it relates to hope in elders with and without cancer.

2. Caregivers' log reports of sleep and activity behaviors of persons with Alzheimer's Disease.

3. Nutritional risk factors of noninstitutionalized elderly.

4. Well-being of elderly women: Rural-urban differences.

5. Dimensions and correlates of fatigue in older adults with rheumatoid arthritis.

6. Let the circle be broken: Health of elderly southern Appalachian widows.

7. Self-care in chronically ill older adults.

8. Quality of life of critically ill elderly patients.

9. Nurses' perceptions of factors involved in the usage of physical restraints with elderly patients in an acute care hospital.

10. Observations and residents' perceptions of the nursing home group dining experience: A qualitative study.

11. An ethnonursing study of the influence of extended caregiving on the health status of elderly Anglo-Canadian wives caring for physically disabled husbands.

12. The meaning of care to geriatric persons living in a long-term care institute.

13. The relationships of nurses' critical thinking ability and patients' self-disclosure to accuracy in assessment of depression in elderly medical patients.

14. The effect of low intensity aerobic exercises on muscle strength, flexibility, and balance among sedentary elderly persons.

15. An exploration of elders' perceptions of power and well-being.

16. The experience of loneliness in adult hospitalized, dying persons.

17. Access to care of adults with chronic illness.

18. Determinate of functional status hospitalization, service use, mortality, and placement among aging network elders: Use of Cox's IMCHB as a nursing framework.

19. Daily hassles, problem solving, and psychological well-being in older adults.

20. The use of a masking signal to enhance the sleep of men and women 65 years of age and older in the critical care environment.

21. The perceived enactment of autonomy scale: Measuring the potential for self-care action in the elderly.

22. The effectiveness of a self-care medication education protocol on the home medication behaviors of recently hospitalized elderly.

23. Functional wellness among older adults: Interface of motivation, lifestyle and capability.

24. Incontinence and coping behaviors of elderly persons: Instrument development.

25. Social environments of adult homes and relapse of residents.

26. Older adults' experiences of health promotion.

27. Older widow's experience of living alone at home.

CARDIAC: 1992

1. Functional health social support, and morale of older women living alone in Appalachia.

2. Elders caring for elders: Risk of abuse and neglect?

3. Interpretation of confusion in the aged: Conflicting models of clinical reasoning among nurses.

4. Images of reconciliation: A philosophic inquiry into the nature of the human being.

5. Visit as method of existential inquiry for nursing: Stories of health from the oldest old.

6. The association of functional status and the use of home care in the last year of life.

7. Construction of elderly people's perceived needs for community-based long-term care.

8. Account-making and the meaning of translocation for elders.

9. Hispanic diabetic elders: Self-care behaviors and explanatory models.

10. Hospitalized elders: Attention deficits and acute confusion.

11. Nurses' and elderly patients' decisions regarding physical restraint.

12. Factors influencing the grief responses of adult daughters after the death of an elderly parent.

13. Family caregiver management of problematic behaviors involving a care receiver with dementia.

14. A comparison of the effect of clinical experiences in two health care settings upon student attitudes toward the elderly.

15. Access to care of adults with chronic illness.

16. Social support: A fieldwork study of adjusting to life in a nursing home.

17. Courage in the chronically-ill elderly: A grounded theory study.

18. Health of adult caregivers of the older person and intergenerational family relationships.

19. Factors which influence the self-medication practices of older women.

20. A descriptive analysis of experiences of personal meanings of life among older adults.

21. The relationship between selected variables and urinary continence status in the elderly.

22. Factors contributing to the level of hope among noninstitutionalized elderly.

CARDIAC: 1993

1. Group generation/community creation among the institutionalized elderly.

2. The relationship among complexity of medication functional ability, and adherence to prescribed medication regimen in the homebound older adult.

3. A psychological autopsy of older adults: Chronic dyspnea and suicidal ideation in elderly men.

4. The effects of demographic and illness severity characteristics and skilled home care on hospital readmission.

5. Intergenerational caregiving: Transition from grandparent to parent.

6. Family health in chronic illness.

7. The moral certainty or uncertainty of nurses regarding end-of-life treatment decisions.

8. Development of a foot care knowledge test for elderly people with diabetes.

9. Urinary incontinence: The relationship between common sense perceptions and self-care behaviors in rural community dwelling older women.

10. Effects of two types of nursing homes on the behaviors of their residents with dementia: A descriptive comparative analysis.

11. The relationship among humor, divergent thinking, and coping with retirement in older adults.

CARDIAC: 1994

1. Development and testing of an instrument to measure emotional loneliness in the elderly.

2. Antecedents and consequences of perceived memory adequacy in elders.

3. Hip fracture recovery in older women: The influence of self-efficacy, depressive symptoms, and state anxiety.

4. Caregiver-Resident interaction at mealtime in an American nursing home.

5. Crafting the quilt: A phenomenological investigation of older women's experience of spirituality.

6. Spirituality in the homebound elderly.

7. Pain behaviors and confusion in elderly patients with hip fracture.

8. Explication of the meaning of reminiscence for the well elderly living in the community.

9. The relationships of self-care agency and self-care actions to caregiver strain as perceived by female family caregivers of elderly parents.

10. Relationships of sleep-wake rhythm, dream experience, human field motion, and time experience in older women.

11. The live experience of caring for a spouse with Alzheimer's disease: An investigation of rural and urban caregivers.

12. The relationship between nursing unit work and structure as it relates to the functional health of elderly patients.

13. Turnover of nurses employed in long-term care facilities: A test of two models.

14. The grief process of older women whose husbands received hospice care.

15. Self-transcendence, health status, and selected demographic variables as determinants of the ability to perform activities of daily living in non-institutionalized older adults.

16. Hope in the elderly: Exploring the relationship between psychosocial developmental residual and hope.

17. Changing nurse aide behavior to decrease learned helplessness in nursing home elders.

18. A theory of elder Chinese-American's conceptions of health promotion and illness prevention: Conformity with nature.

PEDIATRIC ISSUES: 1990

1. Effect of a health promotion program on the self-care agency of children.

2. The relationship of knowledge and health locus of control of early adolescent male to the use of smokeless tobacco.

3. Self-esteem in children with attention deficit hyperactivity disorder.

4. The relationship between family functioning and adolescent substance use.

5. The everyday life experience of three to six-year-old children with comforting possessions.

6. A model of registered intent to stay in Southern California children's hospitals.

7. Effect of perception of seriousness of children's tonsillectomy on family adaptability and cohesion.

8. Pretend play in pre-schoolers with Down Syndrome.

9. Preschoolers' judgments of nurses and nursing activities.

10. Experimental familiarity and social transmission as factors in the development of children's illness-related conceptions.

11. Public portrayal of infant mortality.

12. Families of children with developmental disabilities: A causal model of family adaptation.

13. The relationship of bereaved parent distress, coping, family functioning, cohesiveness, and spousal support with infant death.

14. Differences between colic and non-colic infant performance on the Brazelton neonatal behavioral assessment scale.

15. Parental and economic stress in relation to school age childrens' peer relations and anxiety experiences six years later.

16. The personal experience of developing sexuality in middle childhood.

17. The relationship of constant and intermittent light and state predominance to salivary cortisol in the newborn.

18. Three families' experiences of living with a child diagnosed with Duchenne Muscular Dystrophy.

19. The experience of families when a child is diagnosed with cancer with a favorable prognosis.

20. An exploration of the parental and spousal experiences of fathers/husbands in families of children with chronic illness.

21. Predicting the marginal cost of direct nursing care for newborns.

22. Family function and sibling self-concept of diabetic children: An exploratory study.

23. Young infants' feeding patterns when sick and well.

24. Self-efficacy expectations and self-management in children with asthma.

25. Development of a behavioral observation instrument to identify orientation of the nurse toward parents of hospitalized children.

26. Parental role perceptions: Instrument development.

27. Family adaptation to childhood chronic illness: Family coping style, family relationships, and family coping status–implications for nursing.

28. Parental competence: Determinants of parental involvement with their infants.

29. Premature infant–nurse caregiver interaction.

30. Illness and treatment appraisal processes of healthy and hemophilic boys.

31. Factors influencing toileting behaviors in toddlers.

PEDIATRIC ISSUES: 1991

1. Hypoglycemia in the neonate delivered by elective cesarean section compared to normal vaginal delivery.

2. Perceived stressors and coping strategies of parents with developmentally disabled children.

3. Self-concept and self-care practices of healthy adolescents.

4. The meaning of chronic illness: A phenomenological study of the experience of the chronically ill child and family.

5. Family responses and self-care activities in school-age children with diabetes.

6. Embracing the ugly child within: Life history of an incest survivor.

7. Factors related to self-care agency and self-care practices of obese adolescents.

8. The influence of health status, gender, and trait anxiety on the stress and coping processes of hospitalized, school-age children.

9. A description of the meaning of moral conflict in pediatric nursing practice: Weaving the fabric of choice.

10. Childrens' experience of parental discipline: A picnic spoiled.

11. An exploration of the acquaintance behaviors of pre-school-aged siblings of high-risk hospitalized newborns during their initial meetings.

12. Perceptions of mothers of nurse caring, health status and competence in infant care.

13. Parental role in pediatric intensive care units.

14. Effects of position on oxygenation, heart rate, and behavioral state in the transitional newborn infant.

15. Caring for abused and neglected children on inpatient child psychiatric units: A cross-sectional study.

16. Prediction of breastfeeding attrition: A test of the theory of planned behavior.

17. Determinants of positive health behavior in middle childhood.

18. Treadmill-elicited stepping in low birth weight infants born prematurely.

19. The relationship of lightwave frequency and sleep-wakefulness frequency in well, full-term Hispanic neonates.

20. The relationship between coping dispositions and power components of dependent-care agency in parents of children with special health care needs.

21. The experience of getting well as perceived by adolescents recovering from trauma: A phenomenological perspective.

22. The experience of homelessness viewed through the eyes of homeless school-aged children.

23. Physiologic response of preterm infants during the early initiation of breastfeeding versus bottlefeeding.

24. Correctness of child safety seat usage and rental program participation.

25. The effect of nonnutritive sucking, offered in response to infant-initiated cues, on the activity level of preterm infants.

26. The relationship of clinical status/severity ICU therapy consumption to nursing resource consumption in a pediatric intensive care unit.

27. The epidemiology of Type I diabetes in children 0–14 years of age in Philadelphia.

28. A structured group nursing intervention for girls who have been sexually abused utilizing Roy's Theory of Person as the Adoptive System.

29. Factors affecting premarital sexual intercourse and contraceptive use among rural adolescent females.

30. Future images: An art intervention with suicidal adolescents.

31. The effect of cognitive restructuring and assertion skills training on the self-efficacy and self-care agency of adolescents undergoing hemodialysis.

32. Impact of marital quality and psychological well-being on parental sensitivity for first time mothers and fathers: A nursing study.

33. The relationship of maternal self-concept, depressive symptoms, and social support to the perception of maternal role attainment and premature infant health outcome.

34. Family functioning as perceived by parents of children with attention deficit disorder: A nursing study.

35. Nursing interventions for adolescents in single-parent families: A problem-solving bibliotherapy approach.

36. The relationships among knowledge, perceived accessibility, and practice of contraception of Mexican-American adolescent females.

37. Life events, self-esteem, and powerlessness among adolescents.

38. Premature infant-nurse caregiver interaction.

39. Factors influencing the psychological adjustment of adult children of alcoholics.

PEDIATRIC ISSUES: 1992

1. Relationships of self-care agency, risk-taking, and health risks in adolescents.

2. Becoming pregnant: Perceptions of black adolescents.

3. Chronically ill children's mothers perceptions of environmental variables.

4. Creating paths: Living with a very low birth weight infant.

5. Making the difference: Environmental effects of outcomes of AIDS prevention efforts in the adolescent community.

6. Childhood chronic illness and family hardiness: Integrating a new diagnosis.

7. A projective measure of adult empathy and emotional availability with young infants.

8. A description of the meaning of moral conflict in Pediatric nursing practice: Weaving the fabric of choice.

9. Catching the asthma: Family caring for school-aged asthmatic children.

10. Evaluating the validity and reliability of the pediatric functional independence measure.

11. Effect of crying and non-nutritive sucking on oxygenation in transitional newborn infants.

12. Quality of life: Individual, family, and social correlates in children with hemophilia.

13. Perceptual determinants of early adolescent health promoting behaviors in one Alabama county.

14. Balancing: An expanding concept of health in young adult males.

15. Predictors of self-care in adolescents with cystic fibrosis—A test and explication of Orem's Theories of Self-Care and Self-Care Deficit.

16. Children's fears in cultural perspective: A comparison of Anglo-Americans and Hispanic-Americans combining ethnographic and survey methods.

17. Coping with unplanned childhood hospitalization: Effects of informational interventions on mothers and children.

18. Mother behaviors, infant behaviors, heart rate and rocking within the early mother-infant relationship.

19. An exploratory investigation on the impact of excessive infant crying on the caregiving environment.

20. Occupational and environmental antecedents of young-onset Parkinsons' disease.

21. Caring in families of children with autism.

22. Physiologic response of preterm infants during the early initiation of breastfeeding versus bottle feeding.

23. Formal operations, puberty, and informed decisions.

24. The relationship between sibling death from trauma and children's acquisition of an accurate concept of death.

25. The identification of family system responses to the perceived impact of chronic illness which promote adaptation in a child with chronic illness.

26. Coping behaviors of young children during a chest tube procedure in the PICU.

27. Clinical knowledge of novice and expert nurses caring for a child with a tracheostomy.

28. Adjustment to new parenthood: Relationship among prenatal factors, intrapartal events, and new parent experiences for primiparous mothers and fathers.

29. Increased parental competency by demonstrating newborn behavioral cues.

30. The effects of a perceptual interaction conference on the self-concept of adolescents with sickle-cell anemia.

31. The relationship between self-care agency, self-care and health in the pregnant adolescent.

32. The unbroken cord: The experience of infant relinquishment through adoption.

33. Coping strategies of preschool-aged children hospitalized in a PICU.

34. The meaning of stressful life experiences as described by nine- to eleven-year-old children: A phenomenological study.

PEDIATRIC ISSUES: 1993

1. Child family characteristics and coping patterns of Indonesian families with a mentally retarded child.

2. Development of attachment behaviors in pregnant adolescents.

3. Adolescent motherhood: The human agency perspective.

4. Pregnant adolescent daughter-mother relationships.

5. Conflict management style, clinically assertive behavior, collegial behavior, and job satisfaction in neonatal intensive care unit nurses.

6. On the edge: A naturalistic study of street kids.

7. The relationships among perceived social support, self-esteem, and acculturation in pregnant and non-pregnant Puerto Rican teenagers.

8. The meaning of hope in parents whose infants died from sudden infant death syndrome.

9. Mothers' discipline and punishment of healthy infants.

10. Life histories of adult survivors of childhood polio.

11. Relationships between self-esteem, social support and adolescent hopefulness.

12. Stress and self-esteem in parents of children with attention deficit hyperactivity disorder.

13. The relationship between personal control and codependency in adult children of alcoholics.

14. Seeking safe passage: Health behaviors of pregnant adolescents.

15. An investigation of the relationship between maternal-infant patterns of synchrony during feeding, preterm infant state, and a parent administered state modulation.

PEDIATRIC ISSUES: 1994

1. Very low birthweight infant temperament at six to eight months of adjustment age on family unit health.

2. A test of a breast feeding intention and outcome model.

3. Stress, family social support, and family balance on maternal adaptation in post birth families.

4. Unplanned pregnancy and parenthood in African-American adolescents: Paying for playing.

5. A history of neonatal ethical dilemmas from 1966 to 1985.

6. Moral decision making by parents of infants who have life threatening disorders.

7. Investigation of life change events: Hope, and self-care agency in inner city adolescents.

8. The role of temperament in pediatric pain response.

9. An examination of factors thought to influence observational learning of young mothers from nurses in the neonatal intensive care setting.

10. Authorizing, foregoing, or withdrawing life support: The meaning for parents.

11. Parental perception of family stress in pediatric health crisis: A phenomenological study.

12. A comparison of mothers of young children with Down syndrome and other mothers on selected body image dimensions.

13. Patient-reported injury associated behaviors and life events among injured, ill and well preschool children.

14. A naturalistic study of a small group of street kids.

15. Therapeutic touch and milk letdown in mothers of non-nursing preterm infants.

16. The relationships among perceived social support, uncertainty, and psychological distress in male and female adolescents recently diagnosed with cancer.

17. Self perceived competencies of latency age children as a function of maternal psychosocial adjustment to chronic illness and children's reports of mothering behaviors.

18. State-trait anxiety of women who have previously affected children with chromosome abnormalities and women of advanced maternal age prior to chronic villus sampling.

19. Bulimia nervosa and the family of origin.

20. Infant post-operative pain behaviors and nurses' decision-making.

21. Adolescent resilience following parental death in childhood and its relationship to parental attachment and coping.

22. Social support for African-American adolescent mothers: An exploratory study.

23. The relationship between binge eating severity and degree of obesity in women.

24. Evaluation of the instrument: Adolescent couple communication about dating and contraceptive use for validity and reliability by adolescent girls.

25. The meanings elderly parents of dependent adult children with developmental disabilities give to their long-term parenting experiences.

26. Affecting behavior of mothers when caring for children under five years of age with diarrhea.

27. Behaviors during free play of abused and non-abused preschool aged children in a preschool setting.

28. Staff approaches during episodes of fear in children.

29. Maternal control style in preschool children born at medical risk.

30. Children's self-responsibility health scale: An instrument development.

31. An exploration of relationships among children's pain perspectives, cognitive development, anxiety and previous pain experiences: Implications for nursing.

32. Effect of rocking bed on methadone-exposed infants treated with oral morphine.

33. Maternal discipline approaches: A comparison between children with conduct problems and a non-clinic group.

HIV/AIDS: 1990

1. Validation of nursing's human need theory in persons with HIV infection.

2. Psychosocial responses among persons with human immuno-deficiency virus infection.

3. The effect of community support groups on psychosocial adjustment, uncertainty, and hopelessness on the person infected with HIV.

HIV/AIDS: 1991

1. The relationship between neuropsychological functioning and serum or plasma levels of tumor necrosis factor Alpha in per-

sons at different stages of infection with the human immunodeficiency virus.

2. Predictive model of AIDS related health behavior among intra-
venous drug users.

3. The effect of community support groups on psycho-social adjustment, uncertainty, and hopelessness in persons with the human immunodeficiency virus.

HIV/AIDS: 1992

1. Confronting the medical model: A Hermeneutic view of the
quest for health care by gay men with HIV and AIDS.

HIV/AIDS: 1993

1. Negotiating the journey: A grounded theory study of family/
friend caregiving in the context of AIDS.

2. Self assessment of HIV risk in women: Functional and dysfunctional patterns of assessment.

3. The meaning of grieving for families living with AIDS.

4. Clinical research ethics and pediatric HIV infection.

HIV/AIDS: 1994

1. Educational intervention to increase self-efficacy among Hispanic college students toward prevention of HIV/AIDS.

2. Caring behaviors as reported by persons with the human immunodeficiency virus.

3. Sex, drugs, and T-cells: Symbolic meanings among gay men
with asymptomatic HIV infection.

4. Intimate strangers: AIDS nursing as a contemporary calling: An
ethnographic study.

5. Relationship among hope, perceived health status, and health-promoting lifestyle in HIV seropositive men.

6. An investigation of the relationships among spirituality, perceived social support, death anxiety and nurse's willingness to care for AIDS patients.

7. Guided imagery: A nursing intervention for symptoms related to infection with human immunodeficiency virus.

8. HIV informal caregiving: Role responsibilities and the effect of case management.

9. The impact of nutritional status and HIV disease progression on survival in patients with HIV infection.

10. Becoming a couple infected with HIV.

PULMONARY: 1990

1. The effects of a pulmonary program on dyspnea, self-care, and pulmonary function of patients with chronic obstructive pulmonary disease.

2. Effects of house dust mite educational programs on adult atopic asthmatic clients' adherence, home allergen levels, and symptomatology.

3. The role of cognitive aptitudes in short-term coping and long-term dysfunction in persons with chronic obstructive pulmonary disease.

4. Variables related to functional status in chronic obstructive pulmonary disease.

5. Nutritional patterns of underweight and normal weight patients with chronic obstructive pulmonary disease.

PULMONARY: 1991

1. Dyspnea intensity, psychological distress, anxiety intensity, and inspiratory effort: Effects on ventilator weaning.

2. The effects of positive mental imagery on hope, coping, anxiety, dyspnea and pulmonary function in patients with chronic obstructive pulmonary disease: Tests of a nursing intervention and a theoretical model.

3. Sleep fragmentation oxygen desaturation as etiology of cognitive disability with obstructive sleep apnea.

PULMONARY: 1992

None

PULMONARY: 1993

1. Incremental threshold loading in chronic obstructive pulmonary disease.

2. A nutritional intervention for persons with chronic airflow limitation.

3. Living with asthma: A phenomenological search for meaning.

4. Physiologic and psychosocial attributes of quality of life in lung transplant candidates.

PULMONARY: 1994

1. Effect of upper respiratory infection on the respiratory muscles of breathing in patients with chronic obstructive pulmonary disease.

MEDICAL/SURGICAL: 1990

1. Disease related stressors, social support, illness behaviors, and outcomes among insulin-dependent diabetics.

2. The expression of hunger and appetite by patients receiving total parental nutrition: A descriptive study.

3. The relationship between appraisal processes and coping in middle-aged persons with non-insulin dependent diabetics.

4. Nurse validation of pressure ulcer risk factors.

5. A model for spinal cord injury.

6. Pain and biofeedback.

7. Body image and self-concept in persons with stomas.

8. Development and validation of a predictive model for post-operative complications after a cholecystectomy.

9. Testing of an instrument to measure acceptance of diabetes: Ideas about diabetes revised.

10. The effect of a post-discharge follow-up program on selected outcomes of hospitalized surgical patients.

11. Families coping with serious injury.

12. Perceived social support, basic needs satisfaction, and coping strategies of the chronically ill.

13. Personal meaning of chronic disruption: Living with Lupus.

14. The stress-coping process in kidney transplant recipients and their family members.

15. Predictors of quality of life for adults who have rheumatoid arthritis.

MEDICAL/SURGICAL:　1991

1. Effect of heparin injectate volume on pain and bruising using the Roy Model.

2. Dimensions and predictors of pain in critically ill thoracoabdominal surgical patients.

3. An experimental study of the effects of activity and inactivity on subcutaneous oxygen tension, subcutaneous perfusion and plasma volume.

4. Quality of life after a stroke.

5. Pain, coping, and depression following burn injury.

6. Health conceptions and practices of individuals who have had poliomyelitis.

7. Psychosocial variables and gender as factors in wellness promotion.

8. Client valued outcomes for hip fracture clients in nursing homes.

9. Temporal patterns of bladder, oral, pulmonary artery and rectal temperature in critically ill adults in a surgical intensive care unit.

10. The pain experience, emotions, and self-regulatory behaviors of individuals with rheumatoid arthritis.

11. Selected self-regulatory variables in clients with chronic health problems.

12. Health status, health behavior, multidimensional health locus of control and factors in the development of personal control in individuals with rheumatoid arthritis.

13. Perception of health by persons with a terminal disease: Implications for nursing.

14. Powerlessness: Health beliefs, and compliance in adult diabetics.

15. Anorexia nervosa from sociocultural perspective variables of vulnerability in a university population.

MEDICAL/SURGICAL: 1992

1. Transforming: Patterns of sexual function in adults with insulin-dependent diabetes mellitus.

2. Effect of the arthritis self-help course on arthritis self-efficacy, perceived social support, purpose and meaning in life and arthritis impact.

3. Traumatic brain injury: The family experience.

4. Learned response to long-term spinal cord injury.

5. Patterns of perceived hunger in healthy adults.

6. Effect of increased extracellular calcium and cadmium on human mononuclear phagocytic cells.

7. Self-management compliance and quality of life in chronic hemodialysis patients.

8. A home-based intervention program for family caregivers of dementia patients.

9. Hope, coping, and rehabilitation outcomes in stroke patients.

10. Metropolitan versus nonmetropolitan caregivers of persons with dementia.

11. A methodological study of self-disclosure in chronically ill patients.

12. Health conceptions and practices of individuals who have had poliomyelitis.

13. The effect of normal saline lavage prior to suctioning in adults.

14. A study of power and spiritualilty in polio survivors using the nursing model of Martha E. Rogers.

15. Comparison of the effects of relaxation and music on postoperative pain.

16. Altered bowel elimination among hospitalized elder and middleaged persons.

17. Stress, coping, and perceived social support in chronic hemodialysis patients.

18. Temporal patterns of bladder, oral, pulmonary artery and rectal temperature in critically ill adults in a surgical intensive care unit.

19. Effect of a gum arabic supplement on the nitrogen excretion and serum urea nitrogen concentrations of chronic renal failure patients on a low protein diet.

20. The effect of a diabetes education program: Social support, diabetes knowledge level, blood glucose level, and weight among non-insulin dependent diabetics.

MEDICAL/SURGICAL: 1993

1. Complications and referrals of patients with protein calorie malnutrition.
2. Effectiveness of selected nursing interventions on the conservation of aphasic patients' energy and integrity.
3. Adaptation to spinal cord injury.
4. Risk factors for bone fragility: A longitudinal study.
5. Waiting for a second chance at life: An examination of health-related hardiness, uncertainty, power, and the environment in adults of the kidney transplant waiting list.
6. Psychosocial factors and health status in rheumatoid arthritis: A predictive model.
7. The relationship of diabetic autonomic neuropathy to impaired functional ability in persons with insulin-dependent diabetes mellitus.
8. Relationships between pressure ulcer risk, nursing interventions and pressure ulcer presence.
9. Naturalistic study of the nature, meaning and impact of suffering in people with rheumatoid arthritis.

MEDICAL/SURGICAL: 1994

1. The relationship of psychosocial characteristics of continuous ambulatory peritoneal dialysis patients with the occurrence of infectious complications.
2. Caregiving demands, and coping of spousal caregivers of Parkinson's patients.
3. Maintaining well-being in arthritis: Mediators of the adversive condition.
4. Examination of physiologic responses to endotracheal suctioning techniques.
5. Gender differences in quality of life and social support in persons with chronic fatigue syndrome.

6. Psychosocial factors in peptic ulcer disease for women and men.
7. The relationship of social support to attitudes toward and psychosocial adjustment after ambulatory surgery.
8. Therapeutic touch and in vitro erythropoiesis.
9. A case control study on the cost difference between peripherally inserted central catheters and central venous catheters.
10. Pain experiences of traumatically injured individuals in a critical care setting.
11. Determinants of satisfaction with patient controlled analgesia.
12. Choice behaviors performed by persons with Type II diabetes participating in behavioral analysis with nurses.
13. Mexican-American cultural meanings, expressions, self-care, and dependent care actions associated with experiences of pain.
14. Exercise as a therapeutic intervention in gestational diabetes.
15. The effects of suction catheter insertion on head injured adults.
16. Communication-related responses of mechanically ventilated patients.
17. Predicting central nervous system maturation.
18. The ICU experience: A participant observation patient centered study.
19. The experience of adults with potentially life-threatening conditions in their decision-making regarding treatment options.
20. An acute stressor and the physiological, neuro-endocrine, and immune function in healthy women and women with irritable bowel syndrome.

ONCOLOGY: 1990

1. Marital reciprocal support in the context of cancer.
2. Impact on quality of life and functional status in older adults with non-small cell lung cancer.
3. Physical and psychosocial adaptation, social isolation loneliness, and self-concept of individuals with cancer.

4. A comparative study of loneliness, spiritual well-being and Buberian religiosity in cancer patients.

5. Identifying the needs of caregivers of cancer patients at home.

6. Hope, affect, psychological status and the cancer experience.

7. Spiritual well-being, religiousness, and hope: Some relationships in a sample of women with breast cancer.

8. Attentional fatigue and restoration in individuals with cancer.

9. Family culture, family resources, dependent-care, caregiver burden and self-care agency of spouses of cancer patients.

10. Gynecologic cancer as crisis: Predictors of adjustment.

11. The spiritual health of oncology patients: A comparison of nurse and patient perceptions.

ONCOLOGY: 1991

1. Validation of a nursing diagnosis, alteration in comfort, nausea as experienced by oncology patients receiving chemotherapy.

2. An educational nursing intervention to enhance coping, affective state, and delayed cutaneous hypersensitivity in newly diagnosed malignant melanoma patients.

3. Factors related to body image appraisal associated with receiving treatment for a malignant brain tumor.

4. The experienced body, when taken-for-grantedness falters: A phenomenological study of living with breast cancer.

5. Behavioral correlates of lung cancer pain.

6. Psychosocial adjustment to recurrent cancer.

7. Attentional fatigue and restoration in individuals with cancer.

8. Precancer factors and outcomes of weight loss in adults with lung cancer.

9. Temporal differences in coping, mood and stress with chemotherapy.

10. Identifying meaning in the cancer experience for women with breast cancer.

11. Determinants of anticipatory nausea and anticipatory vomiting in adults receiving cancer chemotherapy: A nursing investigation.

12. A nursing study of empathy from the hospice patients' perspective.

13. Psychosocial correlates of adjustment to breast cancer in marital dyads.

14. The relationship among nursing diagnosis and community agencies and services required for lung cancer patients at discharge.

ONCOLOGY: 1992

1. The impact of surgery on natural killer cell cytotoxicity and tumor metastasis in rats.

2. Childhood cancer stressors and protective factors: Predictors of stress experienced during treatment for cancer.

3. Spiritual well-being, religiousness, and hope among women with breast cancer.

4. Tumor necrosis factor, Interleukin 1, and Interleukin 6 in experimental cancer cachexia.

5. The effects of mental imagery on emotions, immune function and cancer outcome.

ONCOLOGY: 1993

1. Cancer risks of nurses to assess the carcinogenic potential of anitneoplastic drugs.

2. Female nurses' perceptions regarding the severity of facial disfigurement in patients following surgery for head and neck cancer: A comparison based on experience in head/neck oncology.

3. Self-esteem, locus of control, and perceived health status in African-Americans with cancer.

ONCOLOGY: 1994

1. A comparison of ambulatory oncology nursing practice models and their associated differences on health resource utilization.

2. Integrating cancer into a life of mostly lived.

3. A comparison of ambulatory oncology, nursing practice models and their associated differences on health recourse utilization.

4. Experience of breast cancer survivorship: A phenomenological study.

5. The relationship among eudemonestic conception of health, internal cancer, locus of control, hope, and health promoting lifestyle in women with breast cancer.

6. Appraisal, coping responses, social support, and psychosocial adjustment to illness in Irish women receiving chemotherapy.

7. A descriptive study of male caregivers's responses to caring for a family member with cancer.

PSYCHIATRIC NURSING: 1990

1. Patterns of psychological adaptation in death and dying: A causal model and exploratory study.

2. Humanistic caring: Personal influences, coping processes, psychological outcomes and coping effectiveness.

3. Influences of social relationships, illness characteristics, and personality on chronic pain and depression.

4. The relationship between the phenomenon of traumatic injury and the patterns of power, human field motion, esteem and risk taking.

5. The influence of personality type on patient satisfaction with ambulatory health care.

PSYCHIATRIC NURSING: 1991

None

PSYCHIATRIC NURSING: 1992

1. Clinical and economical influences on mental health triage decisions.

2. Family decision making for advanced Alzheimer patients.

3. A descriptive study of widows' grief responses, coping processes and social support within Roy's Adaptation Framework.

4. Bibliotherapy: The experience of therapeutic reading from the perspective of the adult reader.

5. Correlates of attachment behavior and psychological adjustment in persons with the progressive illness multiple sclerosis.

6. Coping with the mental illness of one's spouse.

7. Health-seeking resources and adaptive functioning in depressed and nondepressed adults.

8. Staff and patient opinion on variables of importance to discharge from a mental institution.

9. Factors that influence prevention of intrainstitutional violence.

10. Relationship between self-report of sleep quality and selected electrographic sleep variables in depressed patients and normal controls.

11. The relationship between social support and depression in recovering chemically dependent nurses.

12. Change in co-dependence in health promotion following participation in a program for family members of chemical dependents.

13. Personal power perceptions, need satisfaction, and self-esteem: Theory formation.

14. The process of perspective transformation: Instrument development and testing in ex-smokers and smokers.

15. Relationship of external-rated job performance to self-perceived performance and self confidence.

PSYCHIATRIC NURSING: 1993

1. A relational ontology: The interplay of transcendence spirituality, and community.

2. Variables associated with psychological well-being of family members of trauma patients.

3. War and non-war stressors, family resources, coping and family adaptation among Lebanese families.

4. The relationship between empowerment support, motivation for self-care, mental health self-care, well-being and incest trauma resolution in adult female survivors.

5. A Hermeneutic study of the initial aftermath of a near-death experience.

6. A longitudinal study of the natural and constructed social networks of chronically mentally ill out-patients in relation to treatment retention, re-hospitalization, and psychiatric rehabilitation.

7. Effects of multifamily group treatment on relatives of depressed patients.

8. Development and psychometric characteristics of the spirituality assessment scale.

PSYCHIATRIC NURSING: 1994

1. An examination of the relationship between personal and contextual variables and occupational stress-related depression in nurses.

2. A description and comparison of the cognitive appraisal processes, coping modes, and intervening variables that effect the decision of chemically dependent women in choosing to remain in or drop out of a drug treatment program.

3. The process of escalating behavior in psychiatric patients.

4. A comparison of community-based nurses' and older adults perception of depression and hopelessness.

5. Adherence to breast cancer screening guidelines among African-American women of differing employment status.

6. Analysis of citations underprinting frequently used psychiatric mental health nursing interventions.

7. Family health in the families of the young chronically mentally ill.

8. The relationship between depression and self-care agency in young adult women.

9. An inquiry into the essential meaning of sibling relationships for non-schizophrenic siblings of chronically schizophrenic individuals.

10. The relationship between endorsement of the compensatory model of helping and analytic style among nurses who care for wife abuse victims.

11. To know and to serve: The history of the Pennsylvania Hospital Training school for male nurses of the department for mental and nervous disorders.

12. Perceptual reactance, drug of choice, and pain perception in substance abusers.

13. The experiences of seven nurses who relate with violence-prone psychiatric inpatients.

14. Alcohol recovery and transition to parenthood.

15. The wonder of meaning: A phenomenological understanding of spiritual distress.

16. Relationship between feminine hygiene practices: Body image and self-esteem.

17. Perceived alienation in individuals with Type II schizophrenia.

18. Growing up with a mentally ill parent: A phenomenological study of adult perceptions.

19. A phenomenological study of meaning of life in suicidal older adults.

NURSING EDUCATION/NURSING LEADERSHIP: 1990

1. Similarities and differences in curriculum design characteristics of master's nursing administration curricula.

2. Preretirement planning of female registered nurses.

3. Personal and organizational variables related to the strength of mentoring relationships in nursing.

4. Structuring knowledge: An interpretative analysis of curriculum documents.

5. The effect of level of patient acuity on clinical decision-making by critical care nurses with varying levels of knowledge and experience.

6. The deep connection: An echo of transpersonal caring.

7. Nursing identity: The nursing-medicine relationship.

8. A study of the relationship between selected predictor variables and student performance on the National Council Licensure Examination for registered nurses.

9. Classify home health patients based on nursing resource consumption: Model development and validation.

10. Decisional control in the client–provider relationship: An exploratory investigation in a primary care setting.

11. A definition of scholarship by doctorally prepared nurse faculty.

12. Class of nurse executives' responses to chemically dependent nurses.

13. An evaluation of the nursing work environment.

14. Symbostics in nursing administration.

15. Socialization of new graduate nurses in critical care.

16. Impact of nurse case management on initial hospital discharge of technology assisted youth.

17. Case study of selected critical decisions made by a nurse-owner, nurse manager of a home health practice.

18. A measure of patient data management system effectiveness, development and testing.

19. A study to estimate the shortage of nursing in correctional facilities.

20. Effectiveness and cost efficiency of interventions in health promotion.

21. Economic and work satisfaction determinants of the annual number of hours worked by registered nurses.

22. Care and cultural context of Lebanese Muslims in an urban U.S. community: An ethnographic and ethnonursing study conceptualized within Leininger's theory.

23. A qualitative investigation of rehabilitation nursing care in an inpatient rehabilitation unit using Leininger's theory.

24. Knowledge development in nursing: Emergence of a paradigm.

25. The allocation of community health nursing resources as informed by a moral principle of distributive justice.

26. Mentors and self-reports of professionalism in hospital staff nurses.

27. Locus of control and autonomy of nurses in the hospital setting.

28. A comparison of performance of undergrad clinical and faculty instructors as perceived by senior baccalaureate nursing students.

29. The outcomes of manager turnover in nursing.

30. The lived experience of commitment to nursing as perceived by nurses in a specific environment.

31. Nurse-physician collaboration in the intensive care unit.

32. Identification of non-nursing activities of medical-surgical staff nurses: An observational field study.

33. Relationships among nursing care requirements, selected patient factors, selected nurse factors, and nursing resource consumption in home health care.

34. The relationship between dimensions of a hospital organization: Climate and peer culture, the empowerment of nurses, and client outcomes.

35. A study of the caring behaviors of three core mental health professional groups: Psychiatric mental-health nurses, clinical psychologists and clinical social workers.

36. The effects of imagery abilities and various combinations of mental rehearsal and physical practice on learning a novel, psychomotor nursing skill.

37. The effect of a theory course in nursing administration and a subsequent field experience on the profile of leadership style of students in a master's program in nursing administration.

38. The relationship between planned change and successful implementation of computer-assisted instruction within higher education in nursing as perceived by faculty.

39. The relationship among socialization, empathy, autonomy, and unethical student behaviors in baccalaureate nursing students.

40. Tailoring nursing care to the individual client: An analysis of client-nurse discourse.

41. The use of simulated patients as a teaching methodology for developing baccalaureate students' abilities to make nursing diagnoses.

42. Relationship of organizational and nurse subsystem variables to nursing productivity.

43. Essence of nurses' lived experience of empathy in nurse-patient interactions.

44. Organizational decison-making by chief nurse executives: Participation, influence, and strategies.

45. Orientation to, and perceptions of personal power of nurses who have and have not experienced childhood physical and sexual abuse.

46. Differences in attitude toward computer-based video instructions and learner control choice made by baccalaureate nursing students of sensing and intuitive psychological type.

47. The relationship between faculty research productivity and organizational structure in schools of nursing.

48. A study of the Kaiserwerth Deaconess Institute's nurse training school in 1850–1851: Purposes and curriculum.

49. Trends in ethical and moral issues in nursing, 1900–1985.

50. An interpretive study of role conceptions and career experiences of mid-level hospital nurse administrators.

51. The nurse, empathy and patient satisfaction.

52. Job satisfaction of chairpersons of nursing departments in academe.

53. A critical analysis of the health promotion movement and implications for nursing.

54. The articulation of nurses and indigenous healers in Swaziland: A nursing perspective.

55. A study of the relationship of quality circles to job satisfaction, absenteeism and turnover of nurses and patient satisfaction.

56. A descriptive study of the creation and early development of a holistic health center.

57. Registered nurse academic preparation and organizational structure as predictors of nursing productivity, patient length of stay, and costs.

58. A study of care coordination provided by home health nurses.

59. An interpretive analysis of the moral experience of the critical care nurse.

60. Empathy within the nurse-patient relationship.

NURSING EDUCATION/NURSING LEADERSHIP: 1991

1. Career choice satisfaction and career maturity of baccalaureate nursing students.

2. Uncovering clinical knowledge in expert psychiatric nursing practice.

3. Selected demographic variables, organizational characteristics, role orientation, and job satisfaction among nurse faculty.

4. The relationship between organizational structure and role conflict and role ambiguity in top level nurse administrators.

5. Psychological stress reactions, coping strategies and health promotion lifestyles among hospital nurses.

6. Managing patient care: A substance theory of clinical decision making in home health nursing.

7. Organized nursing in the Silver State: A history of the Nevada Nurses Association.

8. Baccalaureate reentry students: Effects of professional support on role conflict and role transition.

9. Self-Preserving: Patterns guiding the experience of interpersonal conflict for female nursing faculty.

10. Interpreting information: Health care communication among family nurses practitioners, interpreters, and Cambodian refugee patients.

11. Descriptive study of models of discharge planning and case management in California.

12. Nursing intensity: Relationship between predicted and actual nursing resource consumption and the effect on patient outcomes.

13. The effect of a planned walking program on communication performance in patients with Alzheimer's Disease.

14. The impact of an individually tailored nursing intervention on human field patterning in clients who experience dyspnea.

15. Rural home nursing: Barriers and impact.

16. United States Army nurses in China-Burma-India theater of World War II, 1942–1945.

17. Ethical decisions in nursing: The do-not-resuscitate decision.

18. Client and nurse satisfaction in home health: Development of an instrument.

19. Perceived important characteristics of role models in nursing from the nursing faculty's perspectives and from the baccalaureate nursing student's perspectives.

20. Mentors in nursing in the University setting.

21. An investigation of learning styles, effective teaching, and student achievement in the experiential nursing clinical environment.

22. Workplace variables and experienced occupational hazards as predictors of health of specialty nurses.

23. Analysis of the nature and extent of implementation and projected implementation of a model proposed to support professional nursing practice in acute care hospitals.

24. The relationships among psychological hardiness, faculty practice involvement and perception of role stress services.

25. Factors contributing to anticipated turnover among civilian registered nurses employed in U.S. army hospitals.

26. The effect of coping, job flexibility, and social support on the emotional and physical health of dual earner family members.

27. Nurses' perception of nurse-physician collaboration.

28. An analysis of moral judgment in registered nurses: Principled reasoning versus caring values.

29. Relationships between medical condition, nursing condition, nursing intensity, medical severity, and length of stay in hospitalized medical-surgical adults using the Theory of Social Organizations as adaptive systems.

30. Moral reasoning and ethical decision making in baccalaureate nursing students.

31. The experience of culturally diverse nurse-client encounters.

32. Staff nurse perceptions of a positive relationship with an appointed first-line manager who is perceived as a leader.

33. A phenomenological investigation of the meaning of feeling professional in nursing practice.

34. Self-reported and patient reported nonverbal communication and empathy levels of nurses.

35. Membership status in the state nurses association and political involvement and political activity of nurses.

36. A decision-analytic approach to clinical nursing.

37. Relationship of nursing care requirements to pattern of nursing home utilization and total length of nursing home stay.

38. The relationship among a pattern of influences in the organizational environment, power of the nurse, and the nurse's empathic attributes: A manifestation of intergrowth.

39. The relationship between faculty and practice and scholarly productivity of nurse educators in NLN accredited baccalaureate students of nursing.

40. An analysis of motivational variables in RN and baccalaureate nursing students.

41. The effect of a theory course in nursing administration and a subsequent field experience on the profile of leadership style of students in a master's program in nursing administration.

42. The baccalaureate nursing student's experience in psychiatric clinical setting: A phenomenological study.

43. The relationships among socialization, empathy, autonomy and unethical student behaviors in baccalaureate nursing students.

44. Analysis of the relationship among type of caregiving (dyad and system), caregiver and care-recipient characteristics and caregiver burden.

45. Content analysis of peak experiences in nursing practice.

46. Nursing students' perceptions of learning clinical judgment in undergraduate education.

47. The relationship between structure and faculty perception of climate in schools of nursing.

48. The development of an instrument to measure self-perception of intuitiveness of practicing nurses.

49. Ethical decision making by nurse executives.

50. The relationship of head nurse role characteristics, job satisfaction, and unit outcomes.

51. An evaluation of the 1987 Texas Senate Bill 1160: The effectiveness of legislated accountability requirements for nurses.

52. Health and nursing practice behaviors of registered nurses related to completion of health promotion disease prevention course.

53. The effects of problem-solving simulations on critical thinking skills of baccalaureate nursing students.

54. Strategy Management in nursing: A concept analysis.

NURSING EDUCATION/NURSING LEADERSHIP: 1992

1. Adelphi survey to identify attributes deemed necessary for faculty in baccalaureate nursing programs to proclaim clinical competence.

2. Meta-analysis on costing out nursing services.

3. The moral reasoning of nurse practitioners.

4. Patient advocacy among institutionalized employed registered nurses.

5. The gift of self: The meaning of the art of nursing.

6. Nursing war: A philosophical study of the relationship between the profession of nursing and political violence.

7. Pentimento Prixis: Weaving, aesthetic experience to evolve the caring beings of nursing: A dialectic.

8. The deep connection: An echo of transpersonal caring.

9. Finding ways to create connections among communities: An ethnography of urban public health nurses.

10. Narrative and nursing: Issues and original works.

11. Rhetoric or reality: A critical analysis of public involvement in the Western Australian health care system.

12. The influence of an organizational pain management policy on nurses' pain management practices.

13. Influence tactics related to leadership styles of chief nurse executives.

14. Senior nursing students' perception of the relationship between teacher behavior constructs and leader behavior constructs.

15. Systematic evaluation of a nursing intervention: Discharge planning.

16. Collegiality among staff registered nurses: Test of a conceptual model.

17. Ethical decision making among staff nurses: A phenomenological study.

18. The orientation phase of the nurse-client relationship: Testing Peplau's Theory.

19. Selected factors influencing the implementation of a computerized nursing care plan system.

20. A dilemma of caring: Ethical analysis and justification of the nurse refusing an assignment.

21. The relationship of female nurses' experience to empathic concern, perspective taking, cognitive complexity and analytic interactive style.

22. Nurse linkage agents' efforts to facilitate use of a research-based innovation.

23. Self-actualization, locus of control, and self-care agency among registered nurses.

24. A study of the relationship among perceptions of the immediate supervisor's leadership style, work environment and self-efficacy as reported by head nurses.

25. Values hierarchies and influence structures of practicing professional nurses.

26. Self-perception of organizational structure, professional autonomy and job satisfaction of first-line nursing managers.

27. School nursing: A study of the relationships of professional characteristics, professional orientation, the environment, and organizational structure to professional practice and satisfaction.

28. The cognitive structure of clinical expertise.

29. Nursing organizational structures in acute care hospitals.

30. The relationship of social support and success on the NCLEX-RN for academically high-risk students in baccalaureate nursing programs in the Middle Atlantic and New England states and in the District of Columbia.

31. The differences between field dependence/independence and two measurements of clinical judgment ability in senior baccalaureate nursing students.

32. Baccalaureate nursing students' reports of perception of social support obtained and social support desired from faculty while in clinical experience.

33. An investigation of critical constructs in a caring model for nursing education: Early theory development.

34. Hardiness: Its relationships to health burnout in undergraduate nursing students.

35. New hospitals, new nurses, new spaces: The development of intensive care.
36. Integrating nursing research findings into the curriculum.
37. The relationships among managerial performance, environmental factors, and staff nurse job satisfaction.
38. Preceptorships in baccalaureate nursing programs for registered nurses.
39. Forms of knowledge and the use of the representativeness heuristic in clinical inferencing tasks of community health nurses.
40. Identification of justice and care moral orientations from real-life moral conflicts of critical care nurses.
41. Hospital patients and nurses' perceptions of quality.
42. A methodology for teaching observational skills to staff nurses.
43. The effects of computerized problem-solving simulations on critical thinking skills of baccalaureate nursing students.
44. Seed of change: The origin of associate degree nursing at Norfolk State University.
45. Organizational correlates of minority student recruitment and retention in baccalaureate schools of nursing in the Southeastern United States.
46. Strategic management in nursing: A concept analysis.
47. Testing Brooke's Causal Model of Absenteeism on nurses.
48. An analysis of the values influencing the perceptions and behaviors of neonatal nurses in selected ethical dilemmas.
49. Nursing diagnoses and other selected patient factors, nursing interventions, and other measures of utilization and outcomes in home health care.
50. The epistemology and ontology of practicing nurses and nurse reasearchers: A comparative study.

NURSING EDUCATION/NURSING LEADERSHIP: 1993

1. Identification of nursing management diagnoses.
2. Sociolinguistic dimensions of nurse practitioner practice.
3. Untrained nurses toward professional preparation in Montana.
4. Adaptation in family caregiving to the provision of incontinent care.
5. Nursing, science and gender: Florence Nightingale and Martha E. Rogers.
6. Nurses' economic preparation for retirement.
7. Nurses' perceptions of job re-entry.
8. Performing health education and knowledge of health teaching-learning principles in Jordanian baccalaureate nursing students.
9. A study to determine the effectiveness of an interactive video instruction program in teaching registered nurses in clinical settings the process of quality assurance in nursing.
10. The relationship between the research productivity and teaching effectiveness of baccalaureate nurse educators.
11. Effectiveness of nurse extern programs as a recruitment and retention strategy.
12. Influencing role conception and perceived autonomy among RN students in a baccalaureate nursing program.
13. Spiritual well-being of baccalaureate nursing students and nursing faculty and their responses about spiritual well-being of persons.
14. Development of a theoretical model to predict retention on Puerto Rican students enrolled in nursing education programs.
15. Noncognitive predictor of academic success and achievement for generic baccalaureate nursing student.
16. Nurse-patient interaction: Observations of touch.

NURSING EDUCATION/NURSING
LEADERSHIP: 1994

1. Clinical decision-making processes of novice female baccalaureate and associate degree nurses.

2. The phenomenon of biculturalism and stress among ethnic minority nurse faculty.

3. The lived experience on seven graduate nursing students and their teachers.

4. A philosophic inquiry into authoritative knowledge in nursing.

5. The lived experience of nursing students in caring for suffering individuals: A phenomenological analysis.

6. Baccalaureate nursing students and the experience of learning professional nurse caring.

7. Effects of registered nurses' work design on hospital unit culture, quality, and cost of patient care.

8. The short run supply of registered nurses.

9. Relationships between nurse expressed empathy, patient perceived empathy and patient distress.

10. The measurement of professional nursing governance.

11. The relationship between self-efficacy, self-esteem and burnout among nurse middle managers.

12. The relationship of attitude and subjective norms to intention to attend non-mandatory continuing education programs among registered professional staff nurses.

13. Locus of control, self-actualization and self-care agency among registered nurses.

14. An investigation of the relationship of power and empathy in nurse executives.

15. The effect of nursing case management on length of stay and resource consumption.

16. Evaluation of the effectiveness of teaching medication administration to associate degree nursing students using a total quality management framework.

17. Organizational culture and faculty use of empowering teaching behaviors in selected schools of nursing.

18. Sense of coherence, perceptions of stress level, and self-appraisal of health in registered nurse students: A Salutogenic perspective.

19. An analysis of learning styles of black American nursing students.

20. The relationship among faculty expectations, subsequent faculty-student interactions, and students' self-actualization.

21. Critical action research and the changing role of the nurse executive: A case study.

22. Effects of selected stress modifiers on test anxiety in baccalaureate nursing students.

23. The effects of concept mapping on pre-nursing students ability to recall physiological concepts.

24. Survival of the fittest: An ethnography of nurse administrators.

25. Development of a computer tool including interactive video simulation for eliciting and describing clinical nursing judgment performance.

26. Patient integration: Toward a theory of moral development of experienced clinical nurses.

27. Staff nurse perceptions of barriers to research utilization and administrative supports for research in hospitals.

28. Job satisfaction, work excitement and social climate factors related to nurses' intent to stay.

29. The relationship of nurse manager behaviors and characteristics to subordinates' perceptions of the work unit climate.

30. The effects of environmental turbulence on nurse performance.

31. Case management at a community nursing center.

32. Toward a clearer understanding of the art of nursing.

Index